Dietary Resilience Strategies in Older Adults with Physical Disabilities

Eva Ferrarová

Dietary Resilience Strategies in Older Adults with Physical Disabilities

Eating for Independence, Agency and Dignity

palgrave
macmillan

Eva Ferrarová
Faculty of Arts
Charles University
Prague, Czech Republic

ISBN 978-3-032-22185-8 ISBN 978-3-032-22186-5 (eBook)
https://doi.org/10.1007/978-3-032-22186-5

This publication has the financial support of grant no. 23-06348S awarded by The Czech Science Foundation for the grant project "Meanings of food intake in old age", undertaken at the Faculty of Arts of Charles University.

This Palgrave Macmillan imprint is published by the registered company Springer Nature Switzerland AG
The registered company address is: Gewerbestrasse 11, 6330 Cham, Switzerland

Preface

This book presents new research on ageing with disability and changes in dietary practices and resilience among older adults living at home in the Czech Republic. It is primarily an empirical study, but it also has a conceptual contribution that interprets the models and patterns of creating resilience strategies related to food from both an anthropological and a gender perspective.

The book is intended not only for academics but also for professionals working with older adults and policymakers concerned with ageing and old age in relation to food. Questions of dietary resilience in older adults have also been addressed in other scholarly works such as Vesnaver (2011, 2012), Jensen (2019), Nyberg (2018), Shlisky (2017) and Whitelock and Ensaff (2018). This book differs from those studies in that it offers a comprehensive view of dietary resilience among home-dwelling older adults, also taking into account gender and the anthropology of food. Rather than focusing solely on specific diseases, it approaches dietary resilience in a holistic way.

The book is based on research funded by the Czech Science Foundation (GAČR) under project No. GA23-06348S 'Meanings of Food

Intake in Old Age'. The research was conducted in cooperation with the Faculty of Arts, Charles University, and Masaryk University in Brno. It involved both older adults living in their own households and those living in nursing homes, as well as nursing home staff. The focus on food stems from my academic background in the anthropology of food and from the fascination I experienced during the research with how strongly older adults strive to overcome age-related obstacles, such as health limitations, illnesses and disabilities, and how inventive they are in doing so. This was especially true for those living at home, as opportunities for resilience are more restricted in nursing homes, where rigid and standardised institutional structures tend to place older adults in more passive roles. Residents of nursing homes therefore deserve a separate publication.

I am grateful to the Czech Science Foundation, the Faculty of Arts at Charles University and colleagues from Masaryk University for the opportunity to carry out this research. I would also like to thank all the older adults who were willing to answer countless questions, allowed themselves to be photographed and filmed and showed me their refrigerators, pantries and kitchens.

Prague, Czech Republic Eva Ferrarova

Acknowledgements I would like to thank my colleagues from the project *Meanings of Food in Old Age*—Lucie Vidovičová, Marcela Petrová Kafková, Petr Fučík and Martina Němcová from Masaryk University in Brno, as well as Tereza Kroužková from Charles University in Prague.

I am also deeply grateful to all the research participants for generously allowing us to enter their lives.

This book is based on a project funded by the Czech Science Foundation (GAČR) and carried out by a team from Charles University in Prague and Masaryk University in Brno. The project began in January 2023 and is scheduled to conclude in December 2025.

Competing Interests The author has no competing interests to declare that are relevant to the content of this manuscript.

Ethics Approval This study was conducted in accordance with the ethical standards laid down in the 1964 Declaration of Helsinki and its later amendments. Ethical approval was granted by the Ethics Committee of the Faculty of Social Studies, Masaryk University, Brno (Approval No. EKV-2022-014; Date [to be added]).

Data collection and analysis were carried out in compliance with ethical guidelines and approved by the Research Ethics Committee of Masaryk University (Approval No. EKV-2022-014; January 18, 2023).

Informed consent was obtained from all individual participants included in the study. All participants were informed about the purpose of the research, their right to withdraw at any time and the ways in which their data would be used and anonymized.

All team members signed the Researcher's Code of Conduct developed as part of the project *The Meaning of Food in Later Life* (GA23-06348S). The Code is based on the International ICC/ESOMAR Code on Market, Opinion and Social Research and Data Analytics, the SIMAR standards, the Ethical Code of the Czech Sociological Association and the regulations set by the Ethics Committee of Masaryk University.

Contents

About the Author

Eva Ferrarová worked for many years in the public sector before entering academia in 2018. Since then, she has been teaching *Food Anthropology and Gender* and *Food Anthropology*at the Faculty of Arts, Charles University in Prague. Her research explores the cultural meanings of food across diverse social and cultural contexts, with a particular focus on eating practices in later life. She is especially interested in how food, ageing and culture intersect and in the forms of dietary resilience that older adults develop in their everyday lives.

List of Tables

1

Introduction

Abstract This chapter introduces the context, aims and scope of the book, situating it within the demographic and health-related changes affecting older adults. It highlights the rising proportion of older adults, the prevalence of chronic illnesses and functional limitations, and the challenges these pose to everyday food practices. The chapter emphasises dietary resilience as a crucial lens for understanding how older adults adapt their eating behaviours to maintain health, autonomy and cultural continuity. The qualitative research underpinning this book is also presented, detailing its focus on home-dwelling older adults in the Czech Republic, the use of personal narratives and the integration of gender and cultural perspectives. The chapter further outlines the book's structure, guiding the reader through theoretical grounding, age- and health-related dietary transitions, gendered eating patterns, empirical findings and the broader implications for policy and practice. By foregrounding the voices of older adults, the chapter establishes a framework for understanding dietary resilience as a multidimensional phenomenon shaped by biological, social, cultural and psychological factors.

Keywords Older adults · Dietary resilience · Qualitative research · Food practices · Ageing · Gender · Cultural continuity · Health

E. Ferrarová, *Dietary Resilience Strategies in Older Adults with Physical Disabilities*,
https://doi.org/10.1007/978-3-032-22186-5_1

By the year 2070, the global population aged 65 years and over is expected to reach 2.2 billion, thus surpassing the number of children under 18. Meanwhile, the world's population aged 80+ will rise to 265 million as early as the 2030s (World Population Prospect 2024).

The population of the EU countries is projected to increase to 453 million in 2026. In all member states, a marked shift in the age structure toward older age groups is expected, whereas younger age cohorts will decline in number. As a result, the old-age dependency ratio will increase sharply in all the member states over the coming decades.

Life expectancy at birth in the EU is projected to increase from 78.4 years in 2022 to 86.1 years in 2070 for men and from 84.0 years in 2022 to 90.4 years in 2070 for women, with the gender gap in life expectancy continuing to narrow (EU 2024 Ageing Report).

In the Czech Republic, the share of people aged 65+ has been continuously increasing; by the end of 2024, they accounted for one-fifth of the population, compared to 13% in 1993. Since 2006, older adults have outnumbered children under 15, and in December 2024, there were 133 older adults for every hundred children. This ratio is expected to exceed two hundred by 2040. Women aged 65 in 2024 could expect to live another 20.8 years, while men of the same age could expect 17.0 years (Czech Statistical Office 2025).

Most of older adults worldwide suffer from some illness or health limitation. In the Czech Republic, 75% of people aged 65 and older have a long-term illness or health problem. The most common causes of death in this age group are circulatory diseases, cerebrovascular diseases, hypertension and cancer, with other significant causes of death, such as Alzheimer's disease, vascular dementia and diabetes, gaining in importance in recent years (Czech Statistical Office 2022).

Whether independent or not, older adults always need to eat. However, many older people experience reduced appetite, leading to lower food intake and an increased risk of malnutrition. Other problems may include side effects from medication, diminished sensory perception, depression, loss of independence and social isolation, all of which can reduce the attractiveness of food. At the same time, food is one of the few activities that remains present throughout life, making it both a source of vulnerability and resilience.

Human eating behaviour is shaped by biological, economic, psychological and sociocultural factors, and at the same time, it is influenced by individual history and specific circumstances. Food can therefore be either mere fuel for survival or a meaningful event that helps to maintain continuity and dignity in later life. In this context, resilience becomes essential, since the way older people cope with health limitations and changing needs is most vividly reflected in their everyday relationship to food (Merchant et al., 2022). How older adults respond to changes in taste, health constraints, dietary recommendations or social isolation reflects their ability to adopt strategies to maintain meaningful eating practices (Gedrich, 2003). Manifestations of resilience among older adults show how they deal with loss, preserve their identity and remain part of the social world and cultural environment through food.

The study of dietary resilience strategies can thus be used to highlight the everyday mobilisation of resources in later life and to examine how these strategies interact with and influence health-related behaviour (Jensen et al., 2019). An active resilience approach and the maintenance of dietary continuity significantly enhance physical resilience, enabling older adults to better cope with stressors and deteriorating health. Regular and nutritious food is crucial for preventing malnutrition and functional decline, which are common in the elderly population (Norman et al., 2021). Dietary resilience is also closely linked to psychological resilience, as quality food provides both sensory and psychological pleasure in itself (Bédard et al., 2020). Dietary resilience can be understood as maintaining an adequate nutritional state despite dietary challenges (Vesnaver & Keller, 2011).

The social aspects of eating are also important for the overall well-being of older adults and increase the likelihood of active and healthy ageing (Grønning et al., 2018). From the perspective of medical anthropology, it is crucial to examine how older adults' health develops over time within social contexts (Inhorn & Wentzell, 2012; Curtis, 2024). It is therefore necessary to value the subjective accounts of older adults and to regard their personal narratives as key data for understanding their health throughout the life course (Darlington & Scott, 2002).

Food anthropology also provides an essential framework for studying the eating practices of older adults, as it presents food not only as a biological necessity but also as a cultural, social and symbolic phenomenon. For older people, food is closely linked to identity, memory and social relations. Shared meals, traditional recipes and everyday kitchen routines help maintain cultural continuity and social bonds. Moreover, food practices also reveal gender roles and differences in resilience strategies (Counihan & Van Esterik, 2013). Food anthropology thus shows how food becomes a symbolic expression of autonomy and belonging. In doing so, it complements biomedical and nutritional perspectives and provides a more holistic understanding of dietary resilience in later life.

Nevertheless, relatively few scholarly publications comprehensively examine the individual experiences of older adults through their own voices and narratives in relation to eating. This book seeks to fill this gap by applying qualitative research methods that give as much voice as possible to the older adults themselves. In the Czech context, this book represents the first systematic study that integrates food anthropology and gender studies into research on older adults' eating practices, thereby contributing new empirical knowledge from a post-socialist region to the ongoing international discussion.

1.1 Research Aims

The book presents the results of a qualitative study titled 'Meanings of Food Intake in Old Age', funded by the Czech Science Foundation. The research involved the Faculty of Arts at Charles University in Prague and the Institute of Sociology at Masaryk University in Brno. The book provides an empirical analysis and description of dietary resilience strategies that older adults with age-related physical limitations, living in their own homes, develop and use in ways that are meaningful to them. This focus aims to contribute to understanding the significance of food for older adults, including how their body perception influences eating behaviours. At the same time, the research and its findings are framed within a conceptual framework and examined through a gender-sensitive lens.

The research was motivated by three factors: (1) there is still a limited body of scholarly literature that examines the dietary resilience strategies of older adults living at home in depth or systematically; (2) the fact that older adults are affected by illness or disability is rarely part of public discourse, which is necessary given that most older adults experience a decline in health with age; and (3) it is essential to overcome the marginalisation of older adult voices in academic discourse, shifting the focus from talking about them to talking with them and engaging with their individual stories, which should be understood as key data and contextualised within their life course and sociocultural framework. Accordingly, this qualitative study pursued the following objectives: (a) to identify the dietary resilience strategies used by older adults living in their own homes and (b) to explore and describe the key forms of dietary resilience concerning gender and cultural context.

This work focuses on describing how older adults cope with changing life circumstances in the context of declining health and explaining the mechanisms and dietary resilience strategies they employ to adapt to these changing conditions within their eating patterns. Focusing on dietary resilience strategies provides insight into how older adults mobilise resources to create meaningful eating situations (Jensen et al., 2019).

The research questions are therefore as follows:

1. What dietary resilience strategies do older adults with physical illness, disability or limitations, living in their own homes, use to adapt to changing life circumstances?
2. What gender differences emerge in the eating habits of older adults?

The research presented in this book is qualitative and limited by the number of respondents. Therefore, this book does not aim to provide a comprehensive overview of the topic, nor does it offer a complete picture of the dietary resilience of older adults living in their own homes in the Czech Republic. It does not address the development of dietary resilience among older adults living in nursing homes. However, the research is important because approximately 97.2% of people over the age of 66 in the Czech Republic live in their own homes, outside the network of registered facilities (Czech Statistical Office 2025). This book thus focuses on these home-dwelling older adults.

1.2 Structure of the Book

Chapter 2 is devoted to the theoretical grounding of the book's topic, which is crucial in any research, as it connects individual qualitative studies with broader theoretical concepts, thereby enhancing the significance, depth and impact of the studies themselves. It transforms specific data into meaningful insights and helps develop new theoretical contributions. Theoretical grounding is also a key tool for critical analysis and the interpretation of findings. In this spirit, the second chapter of the book provides a conceptual framework for the entire work, offering an overview of relevant theories as well as cultural, psychological, social, environmental and health-related factors that influence ageing and the dietary practices of older adults. Scientific theories that can help anchor older adults' dietary practices and the emergence of resilience mechanisms and strategies are introduced in this chapter.

In the research, I drew on the professional literature and existing models that address the relationships between individual and collective determinants of health, diet and adaptation (Sobal & Bisogni, 2009), as well as on findings from other studies on topics related to health, ageing, diet and adaptive and resilience mechanisms. Existing models allow for linking the broader social context with individual decision-making in health and dietary practices (Schwarzer, 2011; Chen et al., 2021). Addressing questions of ageing and related health limitations in the context of nutrition first requires clarifying which concept of ageing is being examined. The scientific community has not reached a consensus on whether old age should be defined as active, happy, successful, positive, satisfied or otherwise. This terminological diversity is the subject of many discussions—both scientific and public. Given the significance of this definition, it is addressed in a dedicated section of Chapter 2.

In the next section of Chapter 2, I focused on theories of resilience, which underpin much of the current research on ageing. Resilience is seen as a key resource supporting quality of life in old age (Angevaare et al., 2020). Separately, the chapter addresses the cultural framework of the topic because, from the perspective of medical anthropology and food anthropology, the relationship between older adults' health and their cultural adaptation can be understood as a complex interplay of biological, social and cultural factors that mutually influence one another. Health is not merely a biological state of the body but a culturally constructed phenomenon whose meaning, experience and treatment are shaped by specific cultural patterns and power structures (Baer et al., 2013).

Chapter 3 focuses on health- and age-related dietary changes and resilience strategies. In later life, food acquires a significance that goes beyond merely satisfying physiological needs, it becomes a means of social contact, emotional support, preservation of identity and cultural continuity. For many older adults, especially those living alone, food becomes a symbol of life memories, identity and daily meaning (Albuquerque et al., 2021; Wang et al., 2024). Both older adults and professionals also consider food essential for maintaining health, preventing chronic diseases and sustaining independence. The eating practices of older people are influenced by many physiological, physical, psychological and social factors. The symbolic and emotional dimensions of food remain strong even in advanced age. Social environment, psychological resilience and gender also play significant roles.

The first part of this chapter is dedicated to transitions, that is, major changes that come with ageing and affect older adults' eating habits. Specifically, it addresses the significance of retirement, widowhood and deteriorating health, along with the associated changes in diet. At the same time, it is crucial to consider the social situation and changes in the cultural environment. These transitions often entail a loss of daily structure, social interactions and motivation to cook. This, in turn, affects older adults' diets: they cook less, eat more often alone, prefer simple or processed foods and have lower intakes of fruits, vegetables and high-quality proteins (Celidoni et al., 2020). The motivation to eat also decreases, which can simultaneously be a relief and a source of nutritional deficits. The final part of this chapter addresses issues related to motivation.

Chapter 4 focuses on the gender dimensions of dietary patterns and resilience among older adults. Gender plays a vital role in how older adults approach their eating habits and their bodies. Perceptions of the body, shaped by lifelong gender norms, influence daily food choices as well as the relationship with oneself. Gender differences in body perception and eating behaviour are well documented across age groups, and evidence shows that these differences persist into later life. Among older adults, gender-specific patterns often manifest in differing relationships to the body as a source of identity, health and control (Clarke & Korotchenko, 2011).

Gender also plays a significant role in relation to health in later life. Women generally have higher levels of health literacy regarding nutrition and more often seek information about healthy eating, read food labels, consult with doctors about their dietary habits and actively participate in preventive programmes. This enables them to better understand their nutritional needs and adapt their behaviour, for example, in connection with chronic diseases. Women's higher motivation to care for their health provides them with tools to act more purposefully and strategically in terms of nutrition than men (von Bothmer & Fridlund, 2005). This chapter addresses these gendered dietary patterns, the relationship of one's own body to eating and the associated resilience strategies.

Chapter 5 presents the qualitative empirical research that forms the foundation of the entire book and its findings. This chapter includes sections covering the research objectives, methodology, data collection and analysis, as well as a substantial section dedicated to the research results obtained from home-dwelling older adults. The chapter also includes a discussion of the research findings.

Participants in our study had to overcome dietary challenges resulting from major life changes. Declining health or pre-existing disabilities were among these obstacles. Nevertheless, resilient participants were determined to maintain the continuity and level of their eating habits to which they were accustomed and which aligned with social norms. They relied on personal resources related to food, as this was a way to preserve their independence. Personal resources about eating—such as knowledge about food and nutrition, cooking skills, good physical condition and financial availability—facilitated the development of adaptive strategies among participants to overcome their nutritional vulnerabilities.

It was found that changes in older adults' eating habits were primarily related to deteriorating health. The results indicate that most older adults develop either positive or negative resilience strategies. Five areas of strategies were identified: mindful eating and pleasure of eating, adaptation to changes, diversification of food sources, social networking and healthy eating.

Chapter 6 contains the general discussion and conclusions. This chapter summarises the main findings, their implications for future research and potential practical applications. Overall, it shows that the eating habits of older adults and dietary resilience strategies need to be approached from multiple perspectives. The book concludes that relevant public and private organisations should address older adults' nutrition not only from a purely nutritional standpoint but also from anthropological, social and gender perspectives. Competent authorities should recognise the need to support the development of resilient dietary strategies and mechanisms among older adults, as this is one way to ensure a dignified and even joyful old age.

References

Albuquerque RA dos S, Carvalho VA, Filho C de MA, Lemos NFD, Cendoroglo MS (2021) The Meaning of Eating for Community-Dwelling Oldest Old who Live Alone: A Qualitative Study. J Gerontol Geriatr Med 7: 106.

Angevaare MJ, Roberts J, van Hout HPJ, Joling KJ, Smalbrugge M, Schoonmade LJ, Windle G, Hertogh CMPM. Resilience in older persons: A systematic review of the conceptual literature. Ageing Res Rev. 2020 Nov;63:101144. https://doi.org/10.1016/j.arr.2020.101144. Epub 2020 Aug 22. PMID: 32835890.

Baer, H.A., Singer, M., & Susser, I. (2013). Medical Anthropology and the World System: Critical Perspectives. Santa Barbara: Praeger. Retrieved August 16, 2025, from https://doi.org/10.5040/9798400684296

Bédard A., Lamarche P.O., Grégoire L.M., Trudel-Guy C., Provencher V., et al. (2020) Can eating pleasure be a lever for healthy eating? A systematic scoping review of eating pleasure and its links with dietary behaviors and health. PLOS ONE 15(12): e0244292. https://doi.org/10.1371/journal.pone.0244292

Celidoni, M., Dal Bianco, C., Rebba, V., & Weber, G. (2020). Retirement and healthy eating. *Fiscal Studies, 41*(1), 199–219. https://doi.org/10.1111/1475-5890.12196

Chen, E., Lam, P. H., Finegood, E. D., Turiano, N. A., Mroczek, D. K., & Miller, G. E. (2021). The balance of giving versus receiving social support and all-cause mortality in a US national sample. *Proceedings of the National Academy of Sciences, 118*, e2024770118.

Clarke, L. H., & Korotchenko, A. (2011). Aging and the body: A review. *Canadian Journal on Aging, 30*(3), 495–510. https://doi.org/10.1017/S0714980811000274

Counihan, C., & Van Esterik, P. (2013). *Food and culture* (Vol. 367). New York, NY: Routledge.

Curtis A (2024). Health, Culture and Society: The Transformative Role of Medical Anthropology in Global Healthcare. J Anthropology Rep. 7:209. https://doi.org/10.35248/2684-1304.24.7.209

ČSÚ (Czech statistical office), 2022. https://csu.gov.cz/docs/107508/5013f290-d45f-e0a8-7341-6979c9e2ed70/31003422.docx?version=1.0

ČSÚ (Czech statistical office), 2025. https://csu.gov.cz/senior-citizens?pocet=10&start=0&skupiny=31&razeni=-datumVydanicSu

Darlington, Y., & Scott, D. (2002). Qualitative Research in Practice: Stories from the field (1st ed.). Routledge. https://doi.org/10.4324/9781003117025

EU 2024 Ageing report. Economic and budgetary projections EU member states: https://economy-finance.ec.europa.eu/publications/2024-ageing-report-economic-and-budgetary-projections-eu-member-states-2022-2070_en

Gedrich K. Determinants of nutritional behaviour: a multitude of levers for successful intervention? Appetite. 2003 Dec;41(3):231-8. https://doi.org/10.1016/j.appet.2003.08.005. PMID: 14637320.

Grønning, K., Espnes, G., Nguyen, C., Rodrigues, A., Gregório, M., Sousa, R., Canhão, H., & André, B. (2018). Psychological distress in elderly people is associated with diet, wellbeing, health status, social support and physical functioning- a HUNT3 study. *BMC Geriatrics*, 18. https://doi.org/10.1186/s12877-018-0891-3.

Inhorn, M. C., & Wentzell, E. A. (2012). *Medical anthropology at the intersections: Histories, activisms, and futures*. Duke University Press. https://doi.org/10.1215/9780822395478

Jensen T, Grønnow L, Jespersen AP. Eating strategies – a qualitative study of how frail, home-dwelling older people in Denmark develop strategies to form meaningful eating situations. *Ageing and Society*. 2019;39(3):590-608. https://doi.org/10.1017/S0144686X17001076

Merchant RA, Aprahamian I, Woo J, Vellas B, Morley JE. Editorial: Resilience And Successful Aging. The Journal of Nutrition, Health & Aging. 2022;26(7):652-656. https://doi.org/10.1007/s12603-022-1818-4. PMID: 35842754; PMCID: PMC9209635.

Norman K., Haß U., Pirlich M. Malnutrition in Older Adults-Recent Advances and Remaining Challenges. Nutrients. 2021 Aug 12;13(8):2764. https://doi.org/10.3390/nu13082764.

Schwarzer, R., Lippke, S., & Luszczynska, A. (2011). Mechanisms of health behavior change in persons with chronic illness or disability: The Health Action Process Approach (HAPA). *Rehabilitation Psychology, 56*(3), 161–170. https://doi.org/10.1037/a0024509

Sobal J, Bisogni CA. Constructing food choice decisions. Ann Behav Med. 2009 Dec;38 Suppl 1:S37-46. https://doi.org/10.1007/s12160-009-9124-5. PMID: 19787306.

Vesnaver, E., & Keller, H. H. (2011). Social Influences and Eating Behavior in Later Life: A Review. *Journal of Nutrition in Gerontology and Geriatrics, 30*(1), 2–23. https://doi.org/10.1080/01639366.2011.545038

von Bothmer, M. I. K., & Fridlund, B. (2005). Gender differences in health habits and in motivation for a healthy lifestyle among Swedish university students. *Nursing & Health Sciences, 7*(2), 107–118. https://doi.org/10.1111/j.1442-2018.2005.00227.x

Wang X, Qi J, Zhang K, Xie H, Wu X. The joy of eating: how eating experiences enhance the well-being of older adults. Front Public Health. 2024 Sep 9;12:1438964. https://doi.org/10.3389/fpubh.2024.1438964. PMID: 39314795; PMCID: PMC11417023.

World Population Prospects 2024: https://desapublications.un.org/publications/world-population-prospects-2024-summary-results

2

Conceptual Framework

Abstract This chapter presents the study's conceptual framework, aiming to demonstrate how ageing and the food practices of older adults can be understood within their sociocultural context. The introduction discusses fundamental approaches that emphasise the significance of food not only as a biological necessity but also as a cultural and social practice. The subsequent overview of theories and models portrays ageing as a complex experience shaped by biological, psychological, social and cultural factors. The discussion on 'what kind of ageing' highlights the tension between normative ideals of active or successful ageing and critical perspectives that point to their limitations and underline the importance of everyday adaptability. The framework further develops the concept of resilience, understood as a dynamic process that enables older adults to cope with life challenges through inner resources, social ties and cultural practices, including those related to food. The dimension of socioeconomic status illustrates that broader economic and structural factors always condition the ability to maintain dignified and meaningful food practices. The conceptual framework thus provides a solid foundation for empirical exploration of how resilience, socioeconomic status and cultural values intersect in the everyday lives of older adults.

E. Ferrarová, *Dietary Resilience Strategies in Older Adults with Physical Disabilities*,
https://doi.org/10.1007/978-3-032-22186-5_2

Keywords Theories · Models · Ageing · Resilience · Cultural factors · Socioeconomic status

2.1 Introduction

Theoretical grounding is essential in any research, as it connects individual qualitative studies with broader theoretical concepts, thereby enhancing a study's significance, depth and impact. Theory provides deeper meaning to specific findings and situates them within context. Theoretical grounding thus serves as an important tool for critical analysis and interpretation of results.

Research on the dietary practices of older adults requires consideration of cultural, socioeconomic and biological factors which intersect and mutually influence one another. Biological factors are determined by the health status of older adults, which, in most cases, gradually declines with age. The social environment and economic situation shape access to and the quality of food, while cultural adaptation influences how older adults perceive and accept dietary changes, often necessitated by health limitations. These factors affect the shaping of human health over time (Lock & Nguyen, 2010; Kral, 2014; Ulijaszek, 2024).

Our research was based on selected relevant theories and models, which need to be elaborated in order to understand the study itself and its underlying logic as well as to ensure that its findings can be properly validated. Selecting the theoretical foundation drew on scholarly literature and existing models that address the relationships between individual and collective determinants of health, diet and adaptation (Sobal & Bisogni, 2009), as well as on findings from other studies concerning health, ageing, nutrition and adaptive and resilience mechanisms. This approach allowed for the integration of the broader social context with individual decision-making regarding health and dietary practices (Schwarzer et al., 2011; Chen et al., 2021; Castruita et al., 2022).

Ageing is not only a biological stage but is also culturally defined, socially constructed, historically conditioned and influenced by policies (Schlütter & Jensen, 2023; Gilleard, 2025). It must be understood within a cultural framework in terms of beliefs about the body, expressions of pain and gender norms (Laz, 1998; Neves & Petersen, 2025). Ageing should also be considered in terms of how older adults experience it themselves. This anthropological approach values subjective accounts and treats personal narratives as key data for understanding culturally shaped experiences of ageing (Helman, 2007; Loy & Kowalsky, 2024). Ageing should therefore be understood as a culturally and politically constructed life stage, not merely as biological decline. Culturally shared attitudes towards the body, pain, dependency and productivity fundamentally shape individual experiences of ageing (Lamb, 2022).

No single theory can fully explain adaptive mechanisms and strategies across a life course, but their integration allows for a deeper understanding. This chapter presents selected approaches, including resilience theories, the life course perspective, a gender perspective and concepts from medical and food anthropology, which together form the conceptual framework of the research.

2.2 Theories and Models

2.2.1 Life Course Perspective (LCP)

The dietary practices of older adults cannot be understood as isolated everyday behaviours, but rather as processes deeply embedded in an individual's life course and broader cultural and social contexts. Food habits, preferences and possibilities in later life are the outcomes of lifelong experiences, historical events, family traditions and structural conditions that influence not only what people eat, but also how they experience eating. The Life Course Perspective (LCP) provides an important framework here, as it views ageing and health as dynamic, temporally and socially conditioned processes (Elder, 1998; Hutchinson, 2005; Bengtson et al., 2005). The dietary practices of older adults are thus seen not merely as a matter of individual choice, but also as a reflection of embodied history—the bodily inscription of the past—which shapes current possibilities and meanings associated with food. For this reason, research on nutrition and health in later life must be linked with approaches that consider cultural, biographical and structural dimensions, thereby capturing the complex nature of ageing in everyday life.

The Life Course Perspective examines how human health and illness are shaped over time and within social contexts (Elder et al., 2003; Inhorn & Wentzell, 2012; Halfon & Hochstein, 2002), emphasising how life events and experiences influence later health outcomes (Elder et al., 2003), all within changing cultural, historical and social frameworks (Lock & Nguyen, 2010). Huber et al. (2011) highlighted the dynamic nature of health by defining it in terms of its capacity for adaptation and self-management in the face of social, physical and emotional challenges. Their concept is grounded in an epidemiological framework in which health results from individual exposure to multiple risks over the life course.

Although LCP has been applied in many areas of health and human development research, its direct application is not without challenges and has been repeatedly critiqued. One major criticism is LCP's tendency to assume universal developmental trajectories and structurally defined life stages, which may not correspond to cultural realities or individuals' subjective experiences. Janssen (2009) points out that the conceptualisation of life stages often ignores cultural and discursive variability, leading to cultural rigidity and epistemological flattening. Additional criticism comes from Lynch and Danely (2013), who note that anthropology adopted LCP relatively late and without adequate methodological grounding.

While sociology and psychology have developed robust longitudinal methods, anthropology has traditionally relied on ethnography and situated knowledge. The uncritical adoption of LCP can therefore lead to methodological tension or the inappropriate application of theoretical models. Mattingly (2010) further notes that in clinical contexts, rigid application of this theory may conflict with the need for practical and holistic approaches. In settings where trust and culturally sensitive care must be maintained, anthropologists often take a critical stance towards normative developmental models that may disrupt local understandings of health, ageing and adaptation. From the perspective of critical medical anthropology, Baer et al. (2013) highlight that LCP may overlook broader political, economic and structural determinants of health.

Rather than analysing power inequality, poverty or systemic forms of marginalisation, there is a risk that individual development will be understood in isolation and as an individualised process.

2.2.2 Narrative and Phenomenological Approaches

Aware of the limitations associated with applying LCP, this research primarily drew on approaches that respect cultural variability, biographical depth and structural frameworks, with particular emphasis on narrative and biographical perspectives, as well as the phenomenological anthropology of experience. These approaches provided a contextually sensitive understanding of health trajectories in older adults.

The narrative perspective foregrounds interpretation, focusing on how individuals construct their life courses through storytelling and how such narratives reflect and challenge cultural norms (Mattingly, 1998, 2010). The biographical method further allows for the inclusion of subjective variability and individual differences often obscured by universalising theories (Chamberlayne et al., 2000). In medical anthropology, this approach has proven pivotal in examining patients' experiences, their personal biographies and the interplay between individual narratives and the structural conditions of life (Good, 1994), as personal stories constitute essential qualitative data for understanding health across the life course (Hájek et al., 2012).

The phenomenological perspective contributes to a deeper comprehension of the subjective meanings and culturally specific ways people perceive and experience bodily changes and the ageing process. It emphasises embodied experience and the ways in which people navigate these changes within particular cultural and social contexts. This approach is grounded in the understanding that health, illness and ageing are not merely biological states but modes of being in the world, mediated through the body, the senses and everyday practices (van Rhyn et al., 2020). Phenomenology highlights the importance of subjective experience, intersubjectivity and situatedness, capturing how individuals experience their bodies, pain, vulnerability or vitality in interaction with others and their environment (Fernandez, 2020). Such an approach enables health experiences to be understood not simply as deviations from a normative standard but as dynamic aspects of individuals' lived lives. Together, biographical and phenomenological approaches provide the means to grasp ageing and health in their full biographical depth and embodied situatedness.

2.2.3 Psychological Models of Health Behaviour

While narrative and phenomenological approaches emphasise the culturally and bodily embedded experience of ageing, psychological models of health behaviour provide a framework for understanding decision-making processes and health-related behavioural change at the individual level. Health is not a static state nor merely the outcome of individual choice; rather, it is a dynamically shaped process resulting from embodied life histories and the influence of social environments. Within this context, the Health Belief Model (HBM) is frequently employed. It foregrounds cognitive factors at the individual level, including perceived susceptibility to illness, perceived severity, anticipated benefits, perceived barriers to action and self-efficacy, all of which influence health behaviours (Champion & Skinner, 2008). The HBM has proven particularly useful in explaining why older adults engage—or fail to engage—in preventive care, chronic disease management or health screenings. Crucially, the model acknowledges that personal health beliefs are shaped by long-standing structural conditions such as poverty, discrimination, gender norms and health policy (Herrick & Bell, 2020). The concept of structural vulnerability, as articulated by Bourgois et al. (2017), critically extends the HBM framework, enabling its integration within an anthropological perspective.

While HBM highlights cognitive barriers and motivations in older adults, the dynamic Health Action Process Approach (HAPA) is particularly suitable for explaining how seniors gradually adapt their dietary practices over time. Ralf Schwarzer introduced HAPA in the 1990s to overcome some of the limitations of the relatively static HBM. It distinguishes between a motivational phase, in which the intention to change is formed, and a volitional phase, in which the intention is transformed into concrete action (Schwarzer, 1992; Luszczynska & Schwarzer, 2003). The model thus captures the entire process of behavioural change, encompassing not only cognitive variables but also action planning, coping planning and various forms of self-efficacy throughout the different phases of the process (Schwarzer & Renner, 2000). Consequently, HAPA is particularly suitable for designing interventions to promote healthy behaviour, for example, in relapse prevention, dietary habit change, the maintenance of physical activity or chronic disease management (Schwarzer, Lippke & Luszczynska, 2011; Schwarzer, 2016).

2.3 Defining Ageing

Addressing questions of ageing and related health limitations in the context of eating first requires clarification about which form of ageing is being examined. The scientific community has not reached a consensus on whether old age should be defined as active, healthy, productive, successful, positive, satisfying or in other terms (Foster & Walker, 2021). These concepts differ in the roles they attribute to older adults and in the extent to which they incorporate LCP. The diversity of terminology has been the subject of extensive discussion, both within academia and in public debate. Given the significance of this definition, it is addressed in a separate section of this chapter. All these concepts can be understood along a continuum between normative, expert and structural models at one end and subjective, narrative and culturally conditioned models at the other.

2.3.1 Successful Ageing

Rowe and Kahn (1997) defined successful ageing as a combination of disease prevention, the maintenance of high mental and physical capacities, and social engagement. Their model supports the idea that old age is not merely the result of biological decline, but can be significantly influenced by lifestyle factors, including diet and physical activity. However, this approach has been criticised for its static nature: it places too much emphasis on individual control and insufficiently considers historical and cultural contexts, social relationships and structural determinants affecting functioning in old age (Stowe & Cooney, 2015).

Furthermore, Rowe and Kahn overestimated the proportion of older adults who age without disease, as their model often relies on normative standards of 'success'. Critics note that this framework places unrealistic pressure on older individuals who do not perceive themselves—or are not perceived by others—as 'successfully ageing' and marginalises those who do not meet these standards (Rubinstein & Medeiros, 2015). The strength of this approach lies in its emphasis on disease prevention and lifestyle. At the same time, its weakness is its normative assumptions and the unrealistic expectation that most older adults will age free of disease.

2.3.2 Active Ageing

Over the past two decades, active ageing has become a central scientific and political concept of later life in the European Union, serving as a key strategy in response to demographic ageing. Active ageing is dominated by a narrow economic or productivist interpretation that prioritises the extension of working life, but in doing so, it compromises its broader value (Foster & Walker, 2021). This version of successful ageing emphasises physical and mental capacities over social and behavioural aspects.

The concept has been criticised for representing predominantly an expert perspective that does not reflect the actual possibilities, experiences and preferences of older adults themselves. It defines 'activity' according to normative expectations, such as economic productivity or civic engagement, without adequately considering cultural or health-related conditions that may limit these forms of participation (Djurovic et al., 2017). The strength of this approach lies in its connection to policies and strategies addressing demographic change, while its weakness is its narrow productivist framework and its neglect of the cultural and health-related limitations of older adults.

2.3.3 Healthy Ageing

The concept of healthy ageing is multidimensional and complex, which makes monistic definitions problematic. A key contribution of the concept is its emphasis on lifelong interactions between the individual and the environment, adaptation to changing circumstances and supportive structures that enhance health and the capacity to manage ageing (Menassa et al., 2023). Healthy ageing is understood as the preservation of functional abilities that enable individuals to meet their needs and actively contribute to society. Health problems are not central to this framework; rather, the focus is on adaptive processes that shape the life course in later life.

Both the practical application and theoretical validity of the concept face significant criticism. The healthy versus unhealthy ageing dichotomy assumes that the absence of disease and high performance are the norm. This dichotomous framing can stigmatise older adults who face health limitations, which are common in this population, and fails to account for the variability of life experiences and adaptations (Katz & Calasanti, 2015). Furthermore, the concept is criticised for often neglecting the influence of socioeconomic and organisational determinants, such as poverty, access to healthcare, education and social support, despite their fundamental role in shaping individuals' opportunities to experience 'healthy ageing'.

Empirical studies show that the prevalence of 'healthy agers' varies widely, ranging from 4.5% to nearly 50%, depending on the definition used, highlighting the difficulty of operationalising this concept (Depp & Jeste, 2006). Additionally, framing healthy ageing as a moral imperative can serve as a tool of discipline, transferring responsibility onto the individual and diverting attention from the need for institutional support and social justice (Stephens et al., 2015). The concept is strongly oriented towards functional capacities and adaptation across the life course. Its weakness lies in the dichotomous division of 'healthy' and 'unhealthy' ageing, which can stigmatise individuals with illness.

2.3.4 Positive Ageing

The concept of positive ageing is grounded in positive psychology and aims to enhance the wellbeing of older adults through the development of skills and coping strategies for current and future challenges (Bar-Tur, 2021). Its goal is to support the quality of life of older adults by strengthening their life engagement and active participation in society. Research in this area focuses on the relationship between psychological wellbeing, mental and physical health, successful ageing and the benefits of psychological wellbeing for overall health improvement (Bar-Tur, 2021).

Rather than focusing on pathology, the concept emphasises growth opportunities, flourishing and the enhancement of functional capacity in later life. However, it faces criticism for placing excessive emphasis on individual responsibility: problematic ageing may be interpreted as a personal failure (Pocock et al., 2023; Boudiny, 2013). These authors highlight that the 'good citizen' framework in positive ageing implies a moral obligation of the individual and overlooks broader structural determinants of ageing, such as access to healthcare or economic resources. Critics, such as Rudman (2006), warn that failure to meet these normative standards is often perceived as personal failure, which can induce feelings of guilt and exclusion among vulnerable older adults. Additionally, Stephens et al. (2015) argue that without sufficient consideration for socioeconomic conditions, access to healthcare or environmental safety, not all individuals can genuinely have the opportunity to age positively. The strength of the positive ageing concept lies in its emphasis on growth, wellbeing and engagement of older adults in society. Its weakness is its individualistic framework and the moral pressure it places on the individual, regardless of structural conditions.

2.3.5 Productive Ageing

The theory of productive ageing is a framework that emphasises the positive contributions older adults can make to society through various activities, such as work, volunteering and caregiving, providing a comprehensive approach to addressing an ageing workforce (Schulte et al., 2018). Critics of the productive ageing concept argue that it can be a coercive notion with potentially negative consequences for both individuals and society. Key criticisms include its neoliberal implications, which emphasise individual responsibility, self-sufficiency and economic productivity, aligning with market-oriented ideologies (Estes et al., 2001).

The concept also reflects ethnocentric biases, as models of productive ageing often embody Western, middle-class values that may not align with other cultural norms (Katz & Calasanti, 2015). Furthermore, the focus on productivity can overshadow other important aspects of ageing, such as emotional wellbeing, leisure activities or caregiving (Holstein & Minkler, 2003). The framework may also be perceived as overly normative, promoting idealised standards of ageing that not everyone can or wishes to achieve. This can result in the neglect of the needs of more vulnerable older adults, such as those with disabilities or chronic illnesses, and contribute to their marginalisation (Krahn et al., 2015).

2.3.6 Happy Ageing

In recent years, scholarly debate has partially shifted towards the concept of happy ageing, which represents one possible framework for ageing in a meaningful and high-quality manner (Mathews, 2024). This approach emphasises the individual's capacity to define what happiness means and which activities or values bring them fulfilment. The 'happy ageing' theory seeks to understand quality of life in later life as the outcome of subjective preferences, cultural specificities and available structural support. Its application, therefore, entails not only the promotion of individual autonomy but also the creation of conditions that enable people to make choices aligned with their values and capabilities.

At the same time, this model has become subject to critique. Mathews (2024) notes that 'happy ageing' can serve as an appealing alternative to 'productive ageing', but without adequate institutional support, it may place excessive emphasis on individual self-sufficiency. Critics from the field of critical gerontology (e.g., Liang & Luo, 2019) further highlight that 'happy ageing' is culturally conditioned and should not be regarded as a universal norm. Interpretations of happiness can differ substantially across cultural and social groups, yet the concept is often presented as a universally valid ideal. Sarah Lamb (2014) demonstrates that ideals of happy ageing may vary across cultural contexts; for example, in some Indian communities, later life is associated with spiritual withdrawal, and dependence on others may not be viewed negatively. The strength of this approach lies in its focus on subjective happiness, cultural specificity and support for autonomy. Its weakness is its cultural conditionality and the risk of reducing responsibility to the individual in the absence of institutional support.

2.3.7 Narrative and Philosophical Approaches

Narrative gerontology emphasises the significance of the life story and individual interpretations of ageing. According to Randall and McKim (2005), older adults construct a 'poetics of life' in which they seek meaning and continuity despite bodily losses or social expectations. In this framework, ageing is not evaluated according to external criteria (e.g., activity or productivity) but rather according to the internal coherence and authenticity of the life narrative.

Furthermore, authors such as Jan Baars (2012) stress the need to perceive ageing as an ethical and philosophical challenge, where questions of good, authenticity and reconciliation with life gain prominence. Such approaches do not consider old age a deficit phase but a stage of potential growth, integration and deep understanding of oneself and others. The strength of this perspective lies in its respect for the subjective life story, meaning and ethical dimensions of ageing. Its weakness is the limited practical applicability in policy and healthcare contexts.

None of the concepts presented can be understood as a universal or exhaustive explanation of the ageing experience. Each emphasises a different aspect of ageing and has its limitations, particularly regarding the neglect of socioeconomic and cultural conditions. In the context of older adults' eating practices, these diverse frameworks highlight different relevant aspects: disease prevention through diet, the enjoyment of food, eating as a means of social participation or memories and life stories associated with food. It therefore becomes evident that no single model can capture the complexity of later life. A pluralistic approach is essential to understanding the dietary practices of older adults.

2.4 Dietary Resilience

Many contemporary studies on ageing and resilience strategies in eating draw on the concept of resilience, which is regarded as a key resource supporting quality of life in later life (Angevaare et al., 2020). Resilience is increasingly understood as a resource available to all individuals throughout the life course, rather than as an exceptional trait possessed by only a few. Nevertheless, there is still no clear consensus on what resilience precisely entails in later life (Taylor & Carr, 2021).

When resilience is conceived as an internal characteristic, research typically focuses on psychological traits such as inner strength, optimism, flexibility or the ability to maintain a realistic perspective on life circumstances. These traits are often measured using tools such as the Resilience Scale (Wagnild & Young, 1993; Smith et al., 2008). From this perspective, resilience can develop over the life course, particularly as a result of successfully coping with challenging or crisis situations. Increasingly, contemporary approaches emphasise resilience as a dynamic process, that is, as a response to stressors through the utilisation of internal and external resources (Wiles et al., 2012).

Bonanno (2004), based on quantitative data on the loss of a loved one, points to multiple pathways to resilience, including personality hardiness, tendencies towards self-development, specific coping strategies and positive emotions, including humour. Further development of the resilience concept, as described by Tusaie and Dyer (2004), characterises it as the aspiration towards above-average functioning, defined as a dynamic interplay of abilities and traits enabling individuals to overcome difficulties and achieve success despite stress or adverse circumstances. Hildon et al. (2010) further expand this definition, conceptualising resilience as achieving better-than-expected outcomes despite adversity.

In palliative care, patients often balance their struggle with illness by accepting their condition and experiencing personal growth even at this stage of their life (Nakashima & Canda, 2005). Qualitative data also show that resilience helps people appreciate courage and integrity in later life without denying the hardships they face (Nygren et al., 2019). Environmental factors, such as access to healthcare, social support and the ability to care for others, also play a crucial role in the development of resilience even in advanced age (Song & Li, 2019).

Determinants of resilience are today predominantly understood as multifactorial and encompass a wide range of variables at different levels of analysis, including genetic, epigenetic, developmental, demographic, cultural, economic and social factors (Masten, 2021; Ungar, 2021). Empirical examination of these determinants is crucial for effectively developing interventions to promote resilience, considering that resilience can be strengthened at multiple levels: individual, family, community and cultural (Southwick et al., 2014). In theory, the term 'resilience repertoire' is often used, referring to the set of skills, strategies and resources that individuals can employ to overcome adverse life events while also allowing for personal growth and development. This repertoire is dynamic and may vary between individuals and across different life stages or situations (Luthar et al., 2000).

Resilience is a fundamental concept for understanding how older adults cope with the challenges associated with ageing. In the context of eating, it plays a crucial role by enabling older adults to adapt to changes brought about by declining health, mobility limitations or loss of appetite. At the same time, it helps overcome social and economic barriers, such as loneliness, lower income or reduced access to quality food.

2.5 Cultural Meaning of Food

Cultural factors influence the ageing process and the development and form of resilience mechanisms. The theory of cultural adaptation assumes the ability of individuals to adjust to and accept changes in their environment, but the pace of this transition varies from person to person. According to Ward (2022), sociocultural adaptation refers to an individual's ability to 'fit in' a new cultural environment and involves adjusting to different values, norms, traditions, language and social practices. Among older adults, the issue of cultural adaptation becomes particularly visible in dietary practices, which reflect both biological needs and cultural meanings. From an anthropological perspective, the relationship between the health status of older adults and their cultural adaptation can be understood as a complex interplay of biological, social and cultural factors that mutually influence one another, since health is not merely a biological state of the body but a culturally constructed phenomenon whose meaning, experience and treatment are shaped by specific cultural patterns and structures of power (Kleinman, 1980; Singer et al., 2020).

2.5.1 Symbolic Dimension

The exploration of food's cultural role can be grounded in three key concepts derived from the ideas of Claude Lévi-Strauss (1969), Mary Douglas (1966, 1972) and Marvin Harris (1975, 1979, 1985), each of whom offers a unique perspective on the complex ways in which food interacts with social structures and cultural practices. The eating practices of older adults should be examined within the broader cultural meanings attributed to food by both individuals and society. In this regard, Claude Lévi-Strauss's (1969) structuralist approach is particularly inspiring, as it emphasises that food practices are culturally constructed through binary oppositions that remain relevant in later life when health limitations often necessitate significant dietary changes. For older adults, a particular food that once symbolised domestic tradition or festive occasions may, due to dietary restrictions, be reclassified as inappropriate or unhealthy, thus undergoing a symbolic shift into the category of the polluted or forbidden. This process is further supported by Mary Douglas (1966), who highlighted the importance of culturally defined boundaries of purity and impurity in food consumption. Such changes can disrupt the sense of continuity and cultural identity, as dietary practices are not merely biological acts but also a means of expressing belonging to a community and a system of values (Counihan & Van Esterik, 2013).

The diet of older adults is thus an integral part of their collective identity, shared with family and the wider community. When older adults are compelled to consume foods that do not align with their customary practices—for example, liquid or mechanically processed meals lacking distinctive flavours—this can lead to feelings of lost dignity or social isolation. Traditional dishes often function as vital connections to the past and to previous generations, and their absence may weaken this symbolic bond (Sutton, 2001). For older adults, it is therefore essential not only to ensure the nutritional adequacy of their diet but also to preserve the cultural relevance and identity of food practices (Fischler, 1988).

In her seminal work *Purity and Danger* (1966), Mary Douglas emphasised that the categorisation of foods and the rules governing their consumption are not based solely on hygienic or nutritional grounds but carry strong symbolic meanings that reflect the broader cultural and social order. Food—like the body and ritual purity—functions, according to Douglas, as a tool of social organisation, helping to establish and maintain boundaries between what is deemed acceptable and unacceptable. This theory gains particular relevance in the context of older adults' eating practices. Many older adults, especially those in institutional care or with specific dietary restrictions, must forgo dishes that once held profound cultural and personal value. Foods that, for decades, formed part of their identity, family tradition and daily life suddenly become prohibited or modified in ways that render them symbolically 'unclean' (Douglas, 1966). This 'uncleanness' does not stem from biological contamination but from the disruption of a culturally shared order that assigns food specific aesthetic, ritual and moral significance. Douglas stresses that violations of such rules may be perceived as breaches of personal as well as social integrity. Among older adults with disabilities, this effect is often heightened by a sense of lost autonomy: not only does their health condition dictate what they must eat, but they are also deprived of participation in the ritual framework of dining, which is vital for shaping identity, memory and relationships with others (Sutton, 2001).

In this context, food functions as a symbolic boundary between active membership in the community and its weakening or loss. While traditional dishes and modes of consumption help sustain family and cultural continuity, their absence may lead to feelings of social exclusion or symbolic 'uncleanness', in the sense of separation from the shared cultural world (Fischler, 1988).

From the perspective of elder care, it is therefore essential that dietary interventions be understood not only as medical necessities but also as culturally sensitive and symbolically significant processes. Respecting the cultural meanings of food and striving to preserve dining rituals, for example, during festive occasions or through specific traditional dishes, can help maintain identity, dignity and meaningful social inclusion even in circumstances of limited independence.

2.5.2 Materialist Perspective

Whereas Lévi-Strauss and Douglas emphasise the symbolic dimension of food, Marvin Harris offers a different perspective focused on material and ecological determinants. In his works, Harris (1975, 1979, 1985) concentrated on the material and ecological foundations of cultural practices, including dietary habits. He argued that human cultural systems, including food preferences, are not primarily shaped by symbolic meanings or ideologies but by practical needs for survival and adaptation to the environment (Harris, 1979). Eating behaviours, in his view, reflect the optimisation of available resources and the efficiency of energy expenditure.

In the context of older adults' nutrition, Harris's theory can be applied particularly to institutional settings (e.g., nursing homes or long-term care facilities), where meals are often designed to minimise costs and maximise the biological functionality of food. Diets in such contexts are usually structured around physiological requirements, caloric values and nutritional content rather than the cultural preferences of the individual. However, this economic-ecological approach may encounter limitations when it overlooks food's symbolic and identity-shaping dimensions. For older adults, whose lives are marked by greater dependency, loss of autonomy and bodily changes, standardised dietary regimes may become a source of social and psychological alienation. For example, the inability to consume traditional dishes due to dietary or institutional restrictions can lead to the loss of a meaningful relationship with food as a cultural marker (Fischler, 1988; Sutton, 2001).

From the perspective of cultural materialism, these situations can be interpreted as a tension between the infrastructural rationality of the system and the individual's cultural needs. Harris's framework suggests that any long-term sustainable dietary strategies, including those implemented in institutional settings, must take into account not only the biological function of food but also its cultural and social meanings, which contribute to the psychosocial wellbeing of the individual (Harris, 1985). This interpretation carries practical implications: meal planning for older adults should not be based solely on nutritional charts and budgetary calculations, but should also consider cultural customs, memory, sensory continuity and the emotional needs of older adults. Such an approach can help preserve quality of life even under conditions of limited autonomy and health-related dependency.

2.5.3 Religion and Dietary Practices

Religion also plays a significant role in shaping dietary habits and rules, not only on the individual level but also within broader cultural and institutional contexts. Dietary prescriptions often derive from theological, moral or symbolic meanings and regulate not only the types of permitted and prohibited foods but also the ways they are prepared, consumed and timed (Douglas, 1966; Fieldhouse, 1986). For older adults with health limitations, adherence to religious dietary rules takes on particular significance, as food may represent one of the last areas of life in which they can maintain cultural identity, autonomy and dignity. Religious rules shape not only the daily diet but can also be essential for preserving the spiritual wellbeing and identity of older adults, especially during periods of illness, restriction or institutionalisation (Mangels et al., 2010). Health-related limitations (e.g., difficulties with swallowing, diabetes, heart disease or reduced mobility) may, however, complicate the observance of religious dietary rules. In some cases, conflicts arise between religious norms and medically prescribed nutrition, which can lead to psychological distress, anxiety or feelings of guilt if older adults are unable to follow the dietary practices of their faith (Koenig, 2004). Research has shown that respecting spiritual needs in elder care can significantly contribute to improved quality of life and greater satisfaction with care (Puchalski et al., 2014).

2.5.4 Health, Migration and Cultural Adaptation

For older adults, especially migrants or individuals living in culturally different environments, the cultural model of health plays a crucial role, that is, the ways in which various cultures explain the origins of illness, approaches to treatment and expectations of the healthcare system. For example, older people from communities in which health is closely tied to spiritual or family values may interpret their symptoms in entirely different ways. They may prioritise traditional healers or family-based care over biomedical approaches (Helman, 2007).

From an anthropological perspective, poor health can also be understood as a symptom of deeper issues, such as cultural alienation, structural inequality or a lack of culturally sensitive healthcare (Lock & Nguyen, 2010). For instance, when older adults face language barriers or experience insensitive treatment from healthcare staff, this can not only worsen their health but also deepen their social isolation and sense of 'non-acceptance', thereby significantly complicating their cultural integration (Inhorn, 1995).

2.5.5 Cultural Factors Shaping Food Practices in Older Adults

Poor health can lead to limited mobility, making it more difficult for older adults to participate in social activities that could support their integration and adoption of new cultural patterns. Health problems, particularly chronic illnesses, can also increase dependence on family or social services, reducing the scope for autonomous adaptation (Torres, 2006). Furthermore, poor health can affect psychological wellbeing, increasing levels of stress, anxiety or depression, which negatively impacts the ability to learn new cultural strategies (Wu & Penning, 2015). Conversely, good health in older adults contributes to greater social engagement, independence and openness to new experiences.

Cultural factors, such as culinary traditions, cultural identity and religious customs, can significantly strengthen resilience in the food practices of older adults with health limitations. Studies show that traditional foods provide comfort, cultural context and motivation to maintain dietary routines (Plastow et al., 2014). Food represents both individual and collective identity among older adults. How meals are prepared and consumed can serve as expressions of ethnic, national or religious affiliation. For older adults who have maintained specific culinary habits throughout their lives, restrictions on access to these practices can be perceived as a loss of autonomy and cultural continuity (Govindaraju et al., 2018).

Food carries symbolic significance, with certain dishes associated with important life milestones or rituals. As a symbol of these milestones, food is not merely a nutritional item but a cultural marker that conveys emotional and collective meanings (Counihan & Van Esterik, 2013). When these foods are unavailable to older adults, it can lead to a sense of alienation from their cultural heritage (Plastow et al., 2014).

The dietary practices of older adults should be understood as a culturally embedded space of resilience. Food connects memory, identity, relationships and a sense of continuity with the past and the community. Losing the ability to consume traditional or symbolically meaningful foods can lead to feelings of isolation, cultural 'uncleanliness' and loss of dignity, whereas maintaining these practices supports resilience against health limitations, social changes and institutional regulations. A practical implication is that care for older adults should be culturally sensitive, not only attending to nutritional guidelines but also respecting the cultural meanings of food, dining traditions and the spiritual dimension of eating. Such an approach allows older adults to preserve their identity, enhances their psychosocial wellbeing and becomes a key element of a high-quality and dignified life, even under conditions of limited autonomy.

2.6 Socioeconomic Context

Social and economic contexts constitute another crucial framework for understanding the experience of ageing. While the social context illustrates how an individual experiences later life within society, the socioeconomic context reveals the material conditions that enable or constrain this experience (Henriques et al., 2020; Berglund et al., 2016). The social context primarily concerns relationships and society: how the individuals are accepted by others, how they perceive their own place and how identity and status change with advancing age (Nutakor et al., 2023). The economic context encompasses the material and financial conditions that affect quality of life in older adulthood (McMaughan et al., 2020). In practice, these two contexts are deeply intertwined, as social relationships are often mediated by material conditions and economic resources gain significance through social connections.

Food intake is particularly important for meeting the social needs of older adults, because beyond its nutritional significance, food plays a central role in maintaining social connections, emotional wellbeing and cultural identity in later life—factors crucial for sustaining quality of life. For older adults, eating is far more than a physiological necessity, it forms the foundation of social wellbeing (Vesnaver & Keller, 2011; Locher et al., 2009). Food intake deepens social interactions and bonds, provides opportunities for community engagement, helps combat loneliness, supports autonomy and independence and facilitates overcoming social barriers.

Pierre Bourdieu's theory of cultural capital and distinction offers a useful framework for understanding eating practices not only in the context of social class but also in relation to ageing and health limitations. Focused initially on social classes more broadly, Bourdieu's theory acquires additional relevance in later life due to health constraints and institutional conditions. Bourdieu (1984) demonstrated that taste and preferences are not natural or individually chosen but socially constructed categories reflecting an individual's position within the social hierarchy. This perspective is equally applicable to older adults with health limitations whose food choices and consumption practices are shaped by both their health status and their cultural capital, as well as by broader structural conditions.

For older adults with health limitations, the situation can be even more complex: their medical condition may completely override their previous eating habits, thereby disrupting the way they previously signalled their social status culturally. Older adults' eating practices are thus shaped by both structural factors (e.g., availability of specialised diet foods, institutional meals in care facilities) and cultural expectations formed in earlier life. Newton-Clarke et al. (2025) examined how socioeconomic status (SES) affects weight loss in older adults, noting that monotonous or aesthetically unappealing meals in care facilities may negatively impact food intake among higher-class older adults, as such meals conflict with their prior identity shaped by cultural capital (Newton-Clarke et al., 2025).

Influenced by SES, food becomes a tool for both social inclusion and exclusion. Older adults who maintain access to diverse, high-quality or culturally meaningful meals can continue to express their class membership. In contrast, those whose diets are entirely determined by health limitations and institutional rules may experience social declassification, which they perceive through the loss of choice or the inability to engage in 'appropriate' dining (House et al., 1994; Bourgois et al., 2017). Health restrictions often affect not only the type of food consumed (e.g., dietary restrictions, mechanically altered meals) but also the manner of consumption (e.g., assisted feeding, isolated dining in care settings). These changes can negatively impact perceptions of personal dignity and social inclusion (Sidenvall et al., 1996).

Food plays a central role in human society as a cultural and social means of expressing relationships, identity and community belonging. Shared meals function as a ritual act that fosters social cohesion and renews connections within the family and the wider society. In this regard, food becomes an important medium of social bonding, particularly during cultural and religious events such as holidays, birthday celebrations or anniversaries (Douglas, 1972; Fischler, 1988; Higgs & Thomas, 2016). For older adults with health limitations, these eating rituals can be disrupted, weakening social ties and the sense of belonging. The disruption of these rituals is thus not merely a cultural loss but also a loss of socioeconomic status, as older adults are no longer able to occupy their original social role.

Socioeconomic status fundamentally influences not only the type and quality of food but also the ability to maintain social and cultural identity. Food becomes a means of expressing class, cultural capital and social standing, and limitations in diet can lead to feelings of social declassification and loss of autonomy.

2.7 Conclusion

The chapter has shown that understanding the ageing experience requires integrating multiple theoretical and empirical perspectives. The introduction outlined the basic approaches to studying ageing and food, emphasising the sociocultural embeddedness of eating practices. Subsequently, theories and models were presented that allow ageing to be understood not merely as a biological process but as a dynamic and relational experience, closely linked to social structures and cultural norms. The discussion of 'which ageing' highlighted the diversity of approaches, ranging from ideals of active and successful ageing to critical perspectives that emphasise the limitations of these concepts and the significance of everyday practices.

Building on this debate, the section on resilience demonstrates that resilience in later life should be understood as a process developing at the intersection of individual capacities, social support and cultural resources. Food practices represent a concrete domain in which resilience manifests as a tool for adapting to change and maintaining continuity of identity. The perspective of socioeconomic status complements this framework by addressing structural conditions that may support or constrain an individual's ability to maintain dietary autonomy and, consequently, quality of life.

Overall, the chapter emphasises that ageing cannot be reduced to individual biological or psychological factors but is the result of a complex interplay of individual, social and cultural conditions, all of which are concretely reflected in the domain of food and eating practices.

References

Angevaare MJ, Roberts J, van Hout HPJ, Joling KJ, Smalbrugge M, Schoonmade LJ, Windle G, Hertogh CMPM. Resilience in older persons: A systematic review of the conceptual literature. Ageing Res Rev. 2020 Nov;63:101144. https://doi.org/10.1016/j.arr.2020.101144. Epub 2020 Aug 22. PMID: 32835890.

Baars, J. (2012). *Aging and the art of living*. Johns Hopkins University Press. https://doi.org/10.1017/S0714980813000548

Baer, H.A., Singer, M., & Susser, I. (2013). Medical Anthropology and the World System: Critical Perspectives. Santa Barbara: Praeger. ISBN 9781440829154

Bar-Tur L. Fostering Wellbeing in the Elderly: Translating Theories on Positive Aging to Practical Approaches. Front Med (Lausanne). 2021 Apr 9;8:517226. https://doi.org/10.3389/fmed.2021.517226. PMID: 33898472; PMCID: PMC8062922.

Bengtson VL, Elder GH, Putney NM, Coleman PG, Kirkwood TBL. The Lifecourse Perspective on Ageing: Linked Lives, Timing, and History. In: Johnson ML, ed. *The Cambridge Handbook of Age and Ageing*. Cambridge Handbooks in Psychology. Cambridge University Press; 2005:493–501.

Berglund H, Hasson H, Wilhelmson K, Dunér A, Dahlin-Ivanoff S. The Impact of Socioeconomic Conditions, Social Networks, and Health on Frail Older People's Life Satisfaction: A Cross-Sectional Study. Health Psychol Res. 2016 Jun 23;4(1):5578. https://doi.org/10.4081/hpr.2016.5578. PMID: 27403463; PMCID: PMC4926029.

Bonanno, G. A. (2004). Loss, trauma, and human resilience: Have we underestimated the human capacity to thrive after extremely aversive events? *American Psychologist, 59*(1), 20–28. https://doi.org/10.1037/0003-066X.59.1.20

Boudiny K. 'Active ageing': from empty rhetoric to effective policy tool. Ageing Soc. 2013 Aug;33(6):1077–1098. https://doi.org/10.1017/S0144686X120 0030X. Epub 2012 Jul 10. PMID: 23913994; PMCID: PMC3728916.

Bourdieu, P. (1984). *Distinction: A social critique of the judgement of taste.* Harvard University Press.

Bourgois P, Holmes SM, Sue K, Quesada J. Structural Vulnerability: Operationalizing the Concept to Address Health Disparities in Clinical Care. Acad Med. 2017 Mar;92(3):299–307. https://doi.org/10.1097/ACM.000000000 0001294. PMID: 27415443; PMCID: PMC5233668.

Castruita PA, Piña-Escudero SD, Rentería ME, Yokoyama JS. Genetic, Social, and Lifestyle Drivers of Healthy Aging and Longevity. Curr Genet Med Rep. 2022 Sep;10(3):25–34. https://doi.org/10.1007/s40142-022-00205-w. Epub 2022 Sep 26. PMID: 38031561; PMCID: PMC10686287.

Chamberlayne, P., Bornat, J., & Wengraf, T. (2000). *The turn to biographical methods in social science: Comparative issues and examples.* London: Routledge. ISBN 9780415228381

Champion, V. L., & Skinner, C. S. (2008). The Health Belief Model. In K. Glanz, B. K. Rimer, & K. Viswanath (Eds.), *Health Behavior and Health Education: Theory, Research, and Practice* (4th ed., pp. 45–65). Jossey-Bass.

Chen E, Lam PH, Finegood ED, Turiano NA, Mroczek DK, Miller GE. The balance of giving versus receiving social support and all-cause mortality in a US national sample. Proc Natl Acad Sci U S A. 2021 Jun 15;118(24):e2024770118. https://doi.org/10.1073/pnas.2024770118. PMID: 34099550; PMCID: PMC8214686.

Counihan, C., & Van Esterik, P. (Eds.). (2013). *Food and culture: A reader* (3rd ed.). Routledge.

Depp CA, Jeste DV. Definitions and predictors of successful aging: a comprehensive review of larger quantitative studies. Am J Geriatr Psychiatry. 2006 Jan;14(1):6–20. https://doi.org/10.1097/01.JGP.0000192501.03069.bc. PMID: 16407577.

Djurovic, I., Jeremic, V., Bulajic, M. *et al.* A Two-Step Multivariate Composite I-Distance Indicator Approach for the Evaluation of Active Ageing Index. *Population Ageing* 10, 73–86 (2017). https://doi.org/10.1007/s12 062-016-9169-8

Douglas, M. (1966). Purity and Danger. London: Routledge and Kegan Paul. https://doi.org/10.4324/9780203361832
Douglas, M. (1972). *Deciphering a meal*. Daedalus, 101(1), 61–81. https://doi.org/10.2307/20023952
Elder GH Jr. The life course as developmental theory. Child Dev. 1998 Feb;69(1):1–12. PMID: 9499552.
Elder, G.H., Johnson, M.K., Crosnoe, R. (2003). The Emergence and Development of Life Course Theory. In: Mortimer, J.T., Shanahan, M.J. (eds) Handbook of the Life Course. Handbooks of Sociology and Social Research. Springer, Boston, MA. https://doi.org/10.1007/978-0-306-48247-2_1
Estes, C. L., Estes, C., Mahakian, J., & Weitz, T. (2001). A political economy critique of "productive aging". In *A political economy critique of "productive aging"* (pp. 187–200). SAGE Publications, Inc., https://doi.org/10.4135/9781452232676.n9
Fernandez AV. Embodiment and Objectification in Illness and Health Care: Taking Phenomenology from Theory to Practice. J Clin Nurs. 2020 Nov;29(21–22):4403–4412. https://doi.org/10.1111/jocn.15431. Epub 2020 Aug 16. PMID: 32741016.
Fieldhouse, Paul. *Food & Nutrition : Customs & Culture*. London ; Dover, N.H: Croom Helm, 1986.
Fischler, C. (1988). Food, self and identity. *Social Science Information, 27*(2), 275–292. https://doi.org/10.1177/053901888027002005
Foster L, Walker A. Active Ageing across the Life Course: Towards a Comprehensive Approach to Prevention. Biomed Res Int. 2021 Feb 3;2021:6650414. https://doi.org/10.1155/2021/6650414. PMID: 33623785; PMCID: PMC7875625.
Gilleard C. Revisiting the social construction of old age. *Ageing and Society*. 2025;45(3):500–513. https://doi.org/10.1017/S0144686X23000570
Good, B. J. (1994). *Medicine, rationality and experience: an anthropological perspective* (No. 1990). Cambridge University Press.
Govindaraju, T., Sahle, B. W., McCaffrey, T. A., McNeil, J. J., & Owen, A. J. (2018). Dietary Patterns and Quality of Life in Older Adults: A Systematic Review. *Nutrients, 10*(8), 971. https://doi.org/10.3390/nu10080971
Hájek, Martin, Havlík, Martin, Nekvapil, Jiří. Narativní analýza v sociologickém výzkumu: přístupy a jednotící rámec. Sociologicky časopis / Czech Sociological Review, 2012, Vol. 48, No. 2: 199–223
Halfon N, Hochstein M. Life course health development: an integrated framework for developing health, policy, and research. Milbank Q.

2002;80(3):433–79, iii. https://doi.org/10.1111/1468-0009.00019. PMID: 12233246; PMCID: PMC2690118.
Harris, M. (1975). *Culture, people, nature: An introduction to general anthropology*. Crowell.
Harris, M. (1979). *Cultural materialism: The struggle for a science of culture*. Random House.
Harris, M. (1985). *Good to eat: Riddles of food and culture*. Waveland Press.
Helman, C. G. (2007). *Culture, Health and Illness* (5th ed.). Hodder Arnold. https://doi.org/10.1201/b13281
Henriques A, Silva S, Severo M, Fraga S, Barros H. Socioeconomic position and quality of life among older people: The mediating role of social support. Prev Med. 2020 Jun;135:106073. https://doi.org/10.1016/j.ypmed.2020.106073. Epub 2020 Mar 31. PMID: 32243939.
Herrick, C., & Bell, K. (2020). Concepts, disciplines and politics: on 'structural violence' and the 'social determinants of health.' *Critical Public Health, 32*(3), 295–308. https://doi-org.ezproxy.is.cuni.cz/https://doi.org/10.1080/09581596.2020.1810637
Higgs, S., & Thomas, J. (2016). Social influences on eating. *Current Opinion in Behavioral Sciences, 9,* 1–6. https://doi.org/10.1016/j.cobeha.2015.10.005
Hildon Z, Montgomery SM, Blane D, Wiggins RD, Netuveli G. Examining resilience of quality of life in the face of health-related and psychosocial adversity at older ages: what is "right" about the way we age? Gerontologist. 2010 Feb;50(1):36–47. https://doi.org/10.1093/geront/gnp067. Epub 2009 Jun 23. PMID: 19549715.
Holstein, J. A., & Gubrium, J. F. (2011). *Varieties of Narrative Analysis*. SAGE
Holstein, M. B., & Minkler, M. (2003). Self, Society, and the "New Gerontology". *The Gerontologist, 43*(6), 787–796. https://doi.org/10.1093/geront/43.6.787
House, J. S., Lepkowski, J. M., Kinney, A. M., Mero, R. P., Kessler, R. C., & Herzog, A. R. (1994). The social stratification of aging and health. *Journal of Health and Social Behavior, 35*(3), 213–234. https://doi.org/10.2307/2137277
Huber M, Knottnerus JA, Green L, van der Horst H, Jadad AR, Kromhout D, Leonard B, Lorig K, Loureiro MI, van der Meer JW, Schnabel P, Smith R, van Weel C, Smid H. How should we define health? BMJ. 2011 Jul 26;343:d4163. https://doi.org/10.1136/bmj.d4163. PMID: 21791490.
Hutchison, E. D. (2005). The Life Course Perspective: A Promising Approach for Bridging the Micro and Macro Worlds for Social Workers. *Families in Society, 86*(1), 143–152. https://doi.org/10.1606/1044-3894.1886

Inhorn MC. Medical anthropology and epidemiology: divergences or convergences? Soc Sci Med. 1995 Feb;40(3):285–90. https://doi.org/10.1016/0277-9536(94)e0029-r. PMID: 7899941.

Inhorn, M. C., & Wentzell, E. A. (Eds.). (2012). *Medical Anthropology at the Intersections: Histories, Activisms, and Futures*. Duke University Press. https://doi.org/10.1215/9780822395478

Janssen, D. F. (2009). Life Course Staging as Cultural and Subjective Practice: Review, Critique, and Theoretical Possibilities. *Culture & Psychology, 15*(4), 541–560. https://doi.org/10.1177/1354067X09344885

Katz S, Calasanti T. Critical perspectives on successful aging: does it "appeal more than it illuminates"? Gerontologist. 2015 Feb;55(1):26–33. https://doi.org/10.1093/geront/gnu027. Epub 2014 Apr 18. PMID: 24747713; PMCID: PMC4986584.

Kleinman, A. M. (1980). *Patients and Healers in the Context of Culture: An Exploration of the Borderland between Anthropology, Medicine, and Psychiatry*. University of California Press. https://doi.org/10.1525/9780520340848

Koenig HG. Religion, spirituality, and medicine: research findings and implications for clinical practice. South Med J. 2004 Dec;97(12):1194–200. https://doi.org/10.1097/01.SMJ.0000146489.21837.CE. PMID: 15646757.

Krahn GL, Walker DK, Correa-De-Araujo R. Persons with disabilities as an unrecognized health disparity population. Am J Public Health. 2015 Apr;105 Suppl 2(Suppl 2):S198–206. https://doi.org/10.2105/AJPH.2014.302182. Epub 2015 Feb 17. PMID: 25689212; PMCID: PMC4355692.

Kral, M. J. (2014). The Relational Motif in Participatory Qualitative Research. *Qualitative Inquiry, 20*(2), 144–150. https://doi.org/10.1177/1077800413510871

Lamb, E. G. (2022). Health Humanities Baccalaureate Programs in the United States and Canada. *Age, Culture, Humanities, 7*, Article 141350. https://doi.org/10.7146/ageculturehumanities.v7i.141350

Lamb S. Permanent personhood or meaningful decline? Toward a critical anthropology of successful aging. J Aging Stud. 2014 Apr;29:41–52. https://doi.org/10.1016/j.jaging.2013.12.006. Epub 2014 Jan 31. PMID: 24655672.

Laz, C. Act Your Age. *Sociological Forum* 13, 85–113 (1998). https://doi.org/10.1023/A:1022160015408

Lévi-Strauss, C. (1969). *The Raw and the Cooked*. University of Chicago Press.

Liang, J., & Luo, B. (2019). Toward a Discourse Shift in Social Gerontology: From Successful Aging to Harmonious Aging. *Cross-Cultural Gerontology*, 34(1), 1–17. https://doi.org/10.1016/j.jaging.2012.03.001

Locher, J. L., Ritchie, C. S., Roth, D. L., Sen, B., Vickers, C. S., & Vailas, L. I. (2009). Food choice among homebound older adults: Motivations and perceived barriers. *The Journal of Nutrition, Health & Aging, 13*(8), 659–664. https://doi.org/10.1007/s12603-009-0194-7

Lock, M., & Nguyen, V.-K. (2010). *An anthropology of biomedicine*. Wiley-Blackwell. ISBN, 1405110724, 9781405110723.

Loy M, Kowalsky R. Narrative Medicine: The Power of Shared Stories to Enhance Inclusive Clinical Care, Clinician Wellbeing, and Medical Education. Perm J. 2024 Jun 14;28(2):93–101. https://doi.org/10.7812/TPP/23.116. Epub 2024 Jan 16. PMID: 38225914; PMCID: PMC11232909.

Luszczynska, A., & Schwarzer, R. (2003). Planning and self-efficacy in the adoption and maintenance of breast self-examination: A longitudinal study on self-regulatory cognitions. *Psychology & Health, 18*(1), 93–108. https://doi.org/10.1080/0887044021000019358

Luthar SS, Cicchetti D, Becker B. The construct of resilience: a critical evaluation and guidelines for future work. Child Dev. 2000 May-Jun;71(3):543–62. https://doi.org/10.1111/1467-8624.00164. PMID: 10953923; PMCID: PMC1885202.

Lynch, C. A., & Danely, J. (2013). Introduction: Transitions and transformations: Cultural perspectives on aging and the life course. In C. A. Lynch & J. Danely (Eds.), *Transitions and transformations: Cultural perspectives on aging and the life course* (pp. 1–22). Berghahn Books.

MacLeod S, Musich S, Hawkins K, Alsgaard K, Wicker ER. The impact of resilience among older adults. Geriatr Nurs. 2016 Jul-Aug;37(4):266–72. https://doi.org/10.1016/j.gerinurse.2016.02.014. Epub 2016 Apr 4. PMID: 27055911.

Masten, Ann S. (2021).Resilience in Developmental Systems In: Multisystemic Resilience. Edited by: Michael Ungar, Oxford University Press (2021). © Oxford University Press. https://doi.org/10.1093/oso/9780190095888.003.0007

Mathews, G. Beyond 'Productive Aging': An Argument for 'Happy Aging'. *J Cross Cult Gerontol* 39, 213–229 (2024). https://doi.org/10.1007/s10823-023-09475-5

Mattingly, C. (1998). *Healing dramas and clinical plots: The narrative structure of experience.* Cambridge University Press. https://doi.org/10.1017/CBO9781139167017

Mattingly, C. (2010). *The Paradox of Hope: Journeys through a Clinical Borderland* (1st ed.). University of California Press. http://www.jstor.org/stable/ https://doi.org/10.1525/j.ctt1ppw0s

McMaughan DJ, Oloruntoba O and Smith ML (2020) Socioeconomic Status and Access to Healthcare: Interrelated Drivers for Healthy Aging. *Front. Public Health* 8:231. https://doi.org/10.3389/fpubh.2020.00231

Menassa M, Stronks K, Khatmi F, Roa Díaz ZM, Espinola OP, Gamba M, Itodo OA, Buttia C, Wehrli F, Minder B, Velarde MR, Franco OH. Concepts and definitions of healthy ageing: a systematic review and synthesis of theoretical models. EClinicalMedicine. 2023 Jan 12;56:101821. https://doi.org/10.1016/j.eclinm.2022.101821. PMID: 36684393; PMCID: PMC9852292.

Mangels, A. R., Messina, V., & Messina, M. (2010). *The dietitian's guide to vegetarian diets: Issues and applications* (3rd ed.). Jones & Bartlett Learning.

Nakashima, M., & Canda, E. R. (2005). Positive dying and resiliency in later life: A qualitative study. *Journal of Aging Studies, 19*(1), 109–125. https://doi.org/10.1016/j.jaging.2004.02.002

Neves, B., & Petersen, A. (2025). The social stigma of loneliness: A sociological approach to understanding the experiences of older people. *Sociological Review, 73*(2), 362–383. https://doi.org/10.1177/00380261231212100

Newton-Clarke A, Johnson MJ, Nwulu U, Murtagh FEM, Bullock AF. Socioeconomic status and older adult's experiences of weight loss: a qualitative secondary analysis. PLoS One. 2025 Apr 22;20(4):e0321313. https://doi.org/10.1371/journal.pone.0321313. PMID: 40261906; PMCID: PMC12013945.

Nutakor, J. A., Zhou, L., Larnyo, E., Addai-Danso, S., & Tripura, D. (2023). Socioeconomic Status and Quality of Life: An Assessment of the Mediating Effect of Social Capital. *Healthcare, 11*(5), 749. https://doi.org/10.3390/healthcare11050749

Nygren, B., Norberg, A., & Lundman, B. (2019). Resilience and growth in older adults facing end-of-life challenges. *Aging & Mental Health, 23*(3), 385–393. https://doi.org/10.1080/13607863.2017.1348472

Plastow NA, Atwal A, Gilhooly M. Food activities and identity maintenance in old age: a systematic review and meta-synthesis. Aging Ment Health. 2015;19(8):667–78. https://doi.org/10.1080/13607863.2014.971707. Epub 2014 Nov 6. PMID: 25373998; PMCID: PMC4440631.

Pocock Tessa, Alistair Woodward, Janine Wiles, Deborah Raphael & Melody Smith (2023) Diverse approaches to conceptualising positive ageing: A scoping review, Kōtuitui: New Zealand Journal of Social Sciences Online, 18:1, 1–26, https://doi.org/10.1080/1177083X.2022.2090968

Puchalski CM, Vitillo R, Hull SK, Reller N. Improving the spiritual dimension of whole person care: reaching national and international consensus. J Palliat Med. 2014 Jun;17(6):642–56. https://doi.org/10.1089/jpm.2014.9427. Epub 2014 May 19. PMID: 24842136; PMCID: PMC4038982.

Randall, W. L., & McKim, A. E. (2005). Toward a poetics of aging: The links between literature and life. *Narrative Inquiry, 14*(2), 235–260. https://doi.org/10.1075/ni.14.2.02ran

Rowe JW, Kahn RL. Successful aging. Gerontologist. 1997 Aug;37(4):433–40. https://doi.org/10.1093/geront/37.4.433. PMID: 9279031.

Rubinstein RL, de Medeiros K. "Successful aging," gerontological theory and neoliberalism: a qualitative critique. Gerontologist. 2015 Feb;55(1):34–42. https://doi.org/10.1093/geront/gnu080. Epub 2014 Aug 26. PMID: 25161262; PMCID: PMC4986589.

Rudman DL. Positive aging and its implications for occupational possibilities in later life. Can J Occup Ther. 2006 Jun;73(3):188–92. https://doi.org/10.1177/000841740607300305. PMID: 16871860.

Schlütter, M. M., & Jensen, T. (2023). Striving to Belong: Everyday Enactments of Belonging among Older Adults in Greenland. *Anthropology and Aging, 44*(1), 19–36. https://doi.org/10.5195/aa.2023.414

Schulte PA, Grosch J, Scholl JC, Tamers SL. Framework for Considering Productive Aging and Work. J Occup Environ Med. 2018 May;60(5):440–448. https://doi.org/10.1097/JOM.0000000000001295. PMID: 29420331; PMCID: PMC6262835.

Schwarzer, R. (1992). Self-efficacy in the adoption and maintenance of health behaviors: Theoretical approaches and a new model. In R. Schwarzer (Ed.), *Self-efficacy: Thought control of action* (pp. 217–243). Hemisphere Publishing Corp.

Schwarzer, R. (2016). Health Action Process Approach (HAPA) as a Theoretical Framework to Understand Behavior Change. *Actualidades En Psicología, 30*(121), 119–130. https://doi.org/10.15517/ap.v30i121.23458

Schwarzer, R., Lippke, S., & Luszczynska, A. (2011). Mechanisms of health behavior change in persons with chronic illness or disability: The Health Action Process Approach (HAPA). *Rehabilitation Psychology, 56*(3), 161–170. https://doi.org/10.1037/a0024509

Schwarzer, R., & Renner, B. (2000). Social-cognitive predictors of health behavior: Action self-efficacy and coping self-efficacy. *Health Psychology, 19*(5), 487–495. https://doi.org/10.1037/0278-6133.19.5.487

Sidenvall B, Fjellström C, Ek AC. Cultural perspectives of meals expressed by patients in geriatric care. Int J Nurs Stud. 1996 Apr;33(2):212–22. https://doi.org/10.1016/0020-7489(95)00042-9. PMID: 8675381.

Singer, Merrill et al. *Introducing Medical Anthropology : A Discipline in Action.* Third edition. Lanham, Maryland: Rowman & Littlefield, 2020. Print.

Smith BW, Dalen J, Wiggins K, Tooley E, Christopher P, Bernard J. The brief resilience scale: assessing the ability to bounce back. Int J Behav Med. 2008;15(3):194–200. https://doi.org/10.1080/10705500802222972. PMID: 18696313.

Sobal J, Bisogni CA. Constructing food choice decisions. Ann Behav Med. 2009 Dec;38 Suppl 1:S37–46. https://doi.org/10.1007/s12160-009-9124-5. PMID: 19787306.

Song J, Li W. Linkage Between the Environment and Individual Resilience to Urban Flooding: A Case Study of Shenzhen, China. Int J Environ Res Public Health. 2019 Jul 18;16(14):2559. https://doi.org/10.3390/ijerph16142559. PMID: 31323739; PMCID: PMC6678611.

Southwick SM, Bonanno GA, Masten AS, Panter-Brick C, Yehuda R. Resilience definitions, theory, and challenges: interdisciplinary perspectives. Eur J Psychotraumatol. 2014 Oct 1;5. https://doi.org/10.3402/ejpt.v5.25338. PMID: 25317257; PMCID: PMC4185134.

Stephens C, Breheny M, Mansvelt J. Healthy ageing from the perspective of older people: a capability approach to resilience. Psychol Health. 2015;30(6):715–31. https://doi.org/10.1080/08870446.2014.904862. Epub 2014 Apr 29. PMID: 24678916.

Stowe JD, Cooney TM. Examining Rowe and Kahn's Concept of Successful Aging: Importance of Taking a Life Course Perspective. Gerontologist. 2015 Feb;55(1):43–50. https://doi.org/10.1093/geront/gnu055. Epub 2014 Jun 6. PMID: 24906516; PMCID: PMC4986588.

Sutton, D. (2001). *Remembrance of Repasts: An Anthropology of Food and Memory.* Berg Publishers. https://doi.org/10.5040/9781350044883

Taylor MG, Carr D. Psychological Resilience and Health Among Older Adults: A Comparison of Personal Resources. J Gerontol B Psychol Sci Soc Sci. 2021 Jun 14;76(6):1241–1250. https://doi.org/10.1093/geronb/gbaa116. PMID: 32750146.

Torres, S. (2006). Elderly Immigrants in Sweden: 'Otherness' Under Construction. *Journal of Ethnic and Migration Studies, 32*(8), 1341–1358. https://doi-org.ezproxy.is.cuni.cz/https://doi.org/10.1080/13691830600928730

Tusaie, K., & Dyer, J. (2004). Resilience: A historical review of the construct. *Holistic Nursing Practice, 18*(1), 3–8. https://doi.org/10.1097/00004650-200401000-00002

Ulijaszek, S. Nutritional anthropology in the world. *J Physiol Anthropol* 43, 10 (2024). https://doi.org/10.1186/s40101-023-00345-0

Ungar, M. (2021). Multisystemic resilience: Adaptation and transformation in contexts of change. *Oxford University Press*. https://doi.org/10.1093/oso/978 0190095888.001.0001

van Rhyn B, Barwick A, Donelly M. Life as Experienced Within and Through the Body After the Age of 85 Years: A Metasynthesis of Primary Phenomenological Research. Qual Health Res. 2020 May;30(6):836–848. https://doi.org/10.1177/1049732319891132. Epub 2019 Dec 13. PMID: 31830854.

Vesnaver E, Keller HH. Social influences and eating behavior in later life: a review. J Nutr Gerontol Geriatr. 2011;30(1):2–23. https://doi.org/10.1080/01639366.2011.545038. PMID: 23286638.

Vesnaver E, Keller HH, Payette H, Shatenstein B. Dietary resilience as described by older community-dwelling adults from the NuAge study "if there is a will -there is a way!". Appetite. 2012 Apr;58(2):730–8. https://doi.org/10.1016/j.appet.2011.12.008. Epub 2011 Dec 16. PMID: 22200412.

Wagnild GM, Young HM. Development and psychometric evaluation of the Resilience Scale. J Nurs Meas. 1993 Winter;1(2):165–78. PMID: 7850498.

Ward, C. (2022). Critical reflections on sociocultural adaptation. *International Journal of Intercultural Relations, 88*, 157–162. https://doi.org/10.1016/j.iji ntrel.2022.03.010

Wiles JL, Wild K, Kerse N, Allen RES. Resilience from the point of view of older people: 'There's still life beyond a funny knee'. Soc Sci Med. 2012 Feb;74(3):416–424. https://doi.org/10.1016/j.socscimed.2011.11.005. Epub 2011 Dec 14. PMID: 22204841.

Wu Z, Penning M. Immigration and loneliness in later life. *Ageing and Society*. 2015;35(1):64–95. https://doi.org/10.1017/S0144686X13000470

3

Dietary Changes and Resilience in Older Adults

Abstract This chapter examines the impact of physiological, psychological, social, economic and cultural changes on the eating behaviour of older adults, as well as the mechanisms that support their dietary resilience. A literature review shows that health limitations, loss of mobility or sensory functions, retirement, widowhood and social isolation can negatively affect food intake and nutritional quality. At the same time, many older adults actively develop resilience strategies, which include adapting their diet, planning meals, using practical aids, maintaining social contacts and engaging in community activities. Cultural and emotional aspects, such as returning to traditional foods, commensality and mindful eating, play a key role in sustaining identity, meaning in life and a sense of wellbeing. The chapter emphasises that dietary resilience is not merely a matter of adaptation but a dynamic process that interconnects the physical, social and cultural dimensions of older adults' lives, supporting autonomy, dignity and quality of life in old age.

Keywords Dietary resilience · Older adults · Ageing · Nutrition · Social support · Cultural identity

E. Ferrarová, *Dietary Resilience Strategies in Older Adults with Physical Disabilities*,
https://doi.org/10.1007/978-3-032-22186-5_3

3.1 Introduction

One of the most significant variables influencing eating patterns in later life, and central to the development of dietary resilience strategies, is health status. Illness, disability and functional limitations affect not only food intake itself but also related activities, such as food selection, shopping, cooking and setting the table. This chapter focuses on how physiological and physical health changes among older adults shape their everyday eating practices. Among the most notable consequences of these changes are eating difficulties (Nyberg et al., 2018), manifested in problems with processing food in the mouth and swallowing. Such challenges can result in inadequate food and nutrient intake as well as social isolation, triggered by feelings of shame or guilt over being unable to eat 'properly' (Nyberg et al., 2018). Eating difficulties are often compounded by reduced appetite, which may lead to unintentional weight loss (Whitelock & Ensaff, 2018).

Another consequence of physical changes is reduced mobility, which significantly affects access to food. Loss of mobility often prevents older adults from going shopping or even from moving around their own homes without fear or difficulty. Mobility problems also include losing the ability to handle food on the plate or bring it to the mouth (Westergren et al., 2014). Impaired vision further influences food practices, for example, in food preparation and cooking, but also in reading labels and distinguishing food items (Whitelock & Ensaff, 2018). In addition, older adults are often burdened with chronic illnesses associated with other age-related symptoms, such as digestive problems or loss of appetite. Body weight also plays an important role, affecting longevity and quality of life. Obesity in later life represents a significant risk factor for chronic diseases and a considerable societal burden. Delaney and McCarthy (2011) note that the life expectancy of obese individuals at age 40 may be reduced by up to seven years compared to individuals of healthy weight. This is crucial to the discussion of dietary resilience, as resilience involves not only the ability to cope with scarcity but also abundance.

In response to these life changes, some older adults develop strategies and mechanisms of dietary resilience that enable them to cope with new situations while maintaining continuity and dignity (Bonanno, 2009). Taylor and Carr (2021) show that interventions to support resilience across the life course can contribute to successful ageing. Older people maintain resilience primarily through social support and the adoption of adaptive mechanisms (Blieszner & Roberto, 2004). Nygren et al. (2005) identify social support, positive adaptation and setting personal goals as the most common resilience strategies among older adults with health limitations. These include, for example, conscious meal planning, avoiding certain foods and drinks or using simple eating aids. Such practices are important for enabling older adults to adhere to socially perceived norms despite declining health. Food is also understood not only as a nutritional source but as a means of maintaining health and as 'fuel' whose primary purpose is to sustain life (Nyberg et al., 2018). Healthy eating is therefore an integral part of resilience strategies (Vesnaver & Keller, 2011). Equally important are learning and development, which stimulate an active mind, strengthen self-confidence and facilitate the acceptance of change (Hayman et al., 2017). Resilience is also reinforced by self-care (Bolton et al., 2016) and the creation of supportive environments that enable independent living and contribute to a sense of safety (Nygren et al., 2005).

In recent years, scholarly literature has increasingly emphasised the importance of food-related pleasure. For some older adults, this dimension extends beyond eating itself to activities such as meal planning, grocery shopping and cooking (Vesnaver et al., 2012). Closely related to food enjoyment is the concept of mindful eating, which stresses a conscious and attentive approach to food. Mindful eating highlights the processual nature of eating—from food acquisition through preparation to consumption. This approach focuses more on the process than on the outcome, since control over food and the situations surrounding its consumption is crucial for older adults in developing dietary resilience (Vesnaver et al., 2012).

However, broader social, economic and cultural variables also shape the eating practices and resilience of older adults. These include, for example, the transition from regular economic activity to retirement (Sydner et al., 2007) or widowhood, when individuals face reduced financial resources and a loss of companionship, given that eating is both a collective and social activity (Whitelock & Ensaff, 2018).

The eating practices of older adults thus emerge from a complex interplay of biological changes, health limitations, economic shifts, social ties and culturally shaped norms. These variables not only restrict access to food or its consumption but also open space for the development of specific resilience strategies that help to maintain continuity, autonomy and dignity. Importantly, food encompasses not only nutritional value but also includes symbolic and emotional aspects, such as social support and adaptation, self-care and the enjoyment of food and the mindful experience of its preparation and consumption. Dietary resilience, therefore, is not merely a reaction to loss or limitation but also an active strategy for sustaining health, quality of life and social embeddedness in later life. This framework is essential for further exploration of the mechanisms through which older adults respond to changes in their everyday eating.

3.2 Changes

Older age is typically a period of transitions and adaptation to losses. These transitions involve profound and often permanent changes in the lives of older adults that extend to eating practices. Later in life, food represents more than nutrition alone; it serves as a means of expressing identity, preserving dignity and maintaining relationships. Retirement is often the first of the major life transitions, and it has significant implications for the eating practices of older adults.

3.2.1 Retirement and Dietary Changes

Retirement is often the first significant change associated with ageing for older adults. Its effects on physical and mental health vary depending on individual attitudes towards retirement and the reasons behind it. A French study reported that approximately one-third of retirees experience difficulties adapting to certain aspects of retirement, such as reduced income and changes in social roles and expectations (Ogg & Renaut, 2019). Data collected in the Czech Republic by the Czech Statistical Office indicate that nearly half of retirements are early, meaning that a significant group of people leave the labour market prematurely. This may be linked to forced circumstances, including deteriorating health (ČSÚ 2025). Such involuntary exits from employment result in a substantial drop in income and a shift in social role, which, in turn, affects the eating habits of retirees.

Some studies have found a deterioration in eating habits after retirement, such as reduced consumption of fruits and vegetables or non-adherence to dietary guidelines (Lagström et al., 2025). In their analysis, Patriota and Marquez-Vidal (2021) showed that within three years after retirement, people increased their intake of saturated fats, animal proteins and alcohol, while a decrease in vegetable consumption and lower Mediterranean diet scores were observed. The research findings, however, are inconsistent: other authors reported improvements in eating habits, such as better adherence to dietary recommendations, increased consumption of vegetables or fish, or no significant changes in dietary patterns (Celidoni et al., 2020; Lagström et al., 2025). Dietary changes partly depended on sociodemographic factors, but they were also gendered. Using data from the Survey of Health, Ageing and Retirement in Europe (SHARE), Celidoni (2020) demonstrated that the transition to retirement led men to reduce their daily intake of fruits and vegetables and increased their risk of obesity. For women, such changes were insignificant. A Finnish prospective study including women who retired between 2000 and 2007 showed that their adherence to dietary recommendations (particularly for fruit, vegetables and fish) improved compared with women who remained employed (Ali-Kovero et al., 2020).

Thus, the literature suggests that the impact of retirement on diet is not uniform but depends on gender, socioeconomic factors and health status. This variability highlights the crucial role of adaptive strategies and the social context.

3.2.2 Widowhood and Eating Behaviours

Widowhood is a major milestone in the lives of older adults and can be even more significant for older adults with disabilities who find themselves without a supportive partner. Widowhood represents a change in the social and dietary context in which a personal system is embedded. Shifts in these contexts are typically a source of changes in individual eating behaviours (Quandt et al., 1998). Should illness and/or health limitations be present, dietary situations usually worsen following widowhood (Shahar et al., 2001).

Adaptive strategies differ between men and women. Some men learn to cook, whereas others rely on eating out or simple meal preparation. Some find a new partner, which restores a source of food provision (Andersen, 2021). For women widowhood entails a loss of their role and identity as food providers and triggers significant changes in eating habits and personal identity. They stop cooking in their previous style and switch to simpler meals (Stahl & Schulz, 2014), often experiencing social loneliness due to the loss of shared meals. A loss of appetite is well documented in women as a symptom of grief (Shahar et al., 2001). Vesnaver (2016) shows that the loss of shared meals triggers a two-phase process: initially, existing eating patterns are disrupted, and subsequently, women reconstruct a personal dietary system adapted to their individual needs. Longitudinal studies also indicate that widowhood is associated with decreased dietary variety; reduced consumption of fruits, vegetables and red meat; and significant weight loss (Stahl & Schulz, 2014).

Kwon et al. (2006) and Stahl and Schulz (2014) report that recently widowed older men, compared with their married peers, more often experience reduced appetite, skipped meals, lower dietary quality and variety and lower fruit and vegetable intake. They describe a decreased motivation to cook and a tendency to select less healthy foods. Furthermore, reviews confirm that widowed men consume more processed foods, eat alone more frequently and lose their appetite, especially when their partner dies from an illness or at an advanced age. An increasing reliance on purchased meals after a partner's death was also reported by Shahar et al. (2001).

Some of the dietary changes associated with widowhood can lead to shifts in, or even a loss of, a focus on healthy eating (Vesnaver & Keller, 2011). In a prospective cohort study, Williams (2004) found that older adults who became widowed showed a marked increase in unhealthy eating habits, particularly among those experiencing a decline in social oversight. Those whose eating habits did not deteriorate had increased supervision from family members or friends.

Widowhood thus represents a critical moment in which the eating practices of older adults can contribute to worsened health and social isolation. At the same time, however, it can also present an opportunity to develop new dietary resilience strategies, including the engagement of social networks, mindful eating and food source diversification.

3.2.3 Declining Health and Dietary Impact

Adequate nutrition is a fundamental condition for healthy ageing. Nevertheless, advanced age is a predictor of reduced food intake and increased nutritional risk (Payette & Shatenstein, 2005; Bailey et al., 2017). Malnutrition is associated with higher mortality (Lange-Chenier, 2013), institutionalisation (Payette et al., 2000) and lower quality of life (Keller et al., 2017). Appetite often declines with age, leading to smaller portions, reduced motivation to prepare meals and increased reliance on ready-made or processed foods. This phenomenon is referred to as the 'anorexia of ageing' and is linked to the loss of taste buds as well as changes in smell and oral microenvironment (Schiffman, 2018). Age-related malnutrition contributes to decreased functional status, weakened immunity, bone loss, anaemia and a higher risk of hospitalisation (de Sire et al., 2022; Wacka et al., 2024). Worsening health, therefore, significantly affects both eating habits and overall nutritional balance in older adults.

One key issue is the increasing prevalence of obesity, which is associated with a higher incidence of chronic diseases (cardiovascular disease, diabetes, osteoarthritis) and greater physical limitations. In later life, sarcopenic obesity—a combination of muscle mass loss and increased fat tissue—often develops, which reduces physical strength, raises the risk of falls and limits daily independence (Roderka et al., 2020; Dondero et al., 2022). Nutrition in such cases is often sufficient in calories but deficient in high-quality protein and micronutrients.

Significant barriers include limited mobility, which complicates grocery shopping and meal preparation. Older adults, therefore, tend to choose simpler, easily prepared meals or products that do not require complex cooking skills (Govindaraju, 2022; Liu et al., 2015). However, these practical adjustments often lead to a decline in nutritional balance, especially for individuals already experiencing taste, smell or digestive issues.

Physiological changes in the digestive system, such as reduced gastric acid secretion, decreased saliva production, slowed peristalsis and impaired regulation of hunger and thirst, reduce nutrient absorption and increase the risk of iron, vitamin B12 and vitamin D deficiencies (Neri & D'Alba, 2021; Sarafrazi et al., 2021). Oral changes, particularly tooth loss and reduced chewing ability, often result in the avoidance of fibrous or hard foods, further limiting dietary variety.

Another factor is polypharmacy, where the frequent use of multiple medications can affect taste, smell and saliva production or cause nausea. The risk of sensory impairments rises with the number of prescribed medications, with four or more daily medications significantly increasing the likelihood of eating difficulties (Schiffman, 2018).

Declining health thus leads to reduced food intake, which weakens the body and further increases the risk of complications. This process has not only biological but also sociocultural consequences. Oral problems or dietary restrictions may hinder commensality, while dependence on ready-made meals alters the daily cooking rhythm and reduces opportunities to maintain culinary traditions.

These challenges also highlight the need for resilient strategies, including modifying recipes, using tools to facilitate meal preparation, engaging family or community support and strengthening cultural identity by maintaining familiar tastes and eating habits in new forms. The ability to adapt can mitigate the negative impacts of health changes and contribute to healthier, more dignified ageing.

3.2.4 Social Transformations and Eating Patterns

Older adults often face social isolation and changes in their cultural environment in response to changes in health status, retirement or widowhood. These life changes can entail a loss of daily structure, social interaction and motivation to cook. This is reflected in their nutrition: they cook less, eat alone more frequently, prefer simple or processed foods and have a lower intake of fruits, vegetables and high-quality proteins (Celidoni et al., 2020). The motivation to prepare complex meals declines significantly. Without the responsibility of providing meals for family and with a reduction in work obligations, older adults tend to switch to simpler or ready-made meals, which can be both a relief and a source of nutritional deficits.

Conversely, community engagement, strong social ties and psychological resilience support better eating habits. Family support is particularly important, enabling older adults to maintain adequate nutrition despite changing life circumstances. Zhang et al. (2022) demonstrated that neighbourhood connections increase the consumption of fresh foods among older adults, while Whitelock & Ensaff (2018) highlight the health benefits of communal eating.

Changes in dietary patterns due to social isolation, limited financial resources or declining health have significant psychological and functional impacts, mostly negative. A lower intake of nutrient-dense foods, particularly fruits and vegetables, increases the risk of physical decline, reduced mobility and decreased quality of life. Depression and loss of appetite, often triggered by loneliness and social isolation, are additional important factors negatively affecting nutrition. Older adults living alone and eating in solitude more frequently exhibit signs of depression and poorer dietary habits (Sakurai et al., 2021). Poor nutrition combined with depression further increases the risk of losing functional independence, mobility and self-care abilities (Park & Kang, 2024). These findings underline the need for systematic support for healthy eating and social connections among the older population.

Nutrition in older adults is therefore not only a matter of individual preferences or health status, it is fundamentally shaped by social ties, cultural habits and the environment in which they live. Social and community connections also provide opportunities for the development of resilient eating strategies and maintaining the quality of nutrition.

3.3 Dietary Resilience

Changes that accompany ageing often create barriers to food intake (Elsner, 2002). However, not all older adults respond to these changes similarly; only some demonstrate resilience and overcome obstacles related to eating (Vesnaver et al., 2012). Currently, little is known about how and why some older adults are able to adapt to these changes and maintain their eating habits, while others are not.

Dietary resilience in older adults refers to the ability to adapt to age-related changes while maintaining appropriate eating habits, adequate nutrient intake and a sense of control over food-related decisions (Vesnaver et al., 2012; Nygren et al., 2005). These strategies include practical approaches, such as adjusting diet, using aids for meal preparation and consumption or modifying shopping routines, as well as psychological and social aspects like maintaining social connections, preserving cultural identity through traditional foods or developing mindful eating practices (Plastow et al., 2015; Wang et al., 2024).

Studying these strategies is important because it demonstrates how older adults can address the nutritional risks and social challenges associated with loneliness, health limitations or changes in domestic and cultural environments (Blieszner & Roberto, 2004; Taylor & Carr, 2021). Understanding the mechanisms of dietary resilience provides valuable insights for interventions, supporting healthy and happy ageing and planning programmes aimed at maintaining autonomy, wellbeing and quality of life for older adults (Southwick et al., 2014).

3.3.1 Motivation and Context

The goal of resilient eating behaviour in older adults is to seek continuity and improve or maintain health, dignity and independence (Vesnaver et al., 2012). The development of this behaviour supports the notion that older adults strive to maintain a stable lifestyle and adapt it to new life situations based on their life experiences (Atchley, 1971). Normative eating behaviour, associated with adequate energy and nutrient intake, should be assessed in relation to the desire for independence (Nyberg et al., 2018). A crucial element of resilience is also cognitive flexibility, which manifests primarily as adaptive thinking; that is, older adults are open to new experiences and willing to change perspectives or approaches when facing new challenges. Cognitive flexibility also entails problem-solving abilities that help them to cope more effectively with obstacles (Hoare, 2021).

According to Vesnaver (2012), dietary resilience represents the development and use of adaptive strategies, with food-related activities holding personal significance for older adults because they play a symbolic role in how adults perceive themselves as individuals, as members of their family and as members of society (Plastow et al., 2015). Engagement in meaningful activities is essential for older adults to maintain autonomy and to preserve personal identity (Phinney et al., 2007). Moreover, qualitative research shows that older adults demonstrate resilience not only by adapting their diet but also by adjusting shopping and eating routines to maintain autonomy and social participation. Recent studies confirm that social capital significantly contributes to maintaining dietary stability and a sense of identity in older adults (Wills & Dickinson, 2023).

Food-related identity often forms early in life and persists over time (Plastow et al., 2015). Declining health, loss of functional abilities or the consequences of illness can threaten dietary identity. For some individuals, this leads to a crisis of self-concept, while others adapt and apply resilient strategies (Plastow et al., 2015). The resilience mechanisms that an individual develops depend on his/her personal history as well as his/her cultural and social identity (Leahy, 2023). Culture and social environment play a significant role in shaping dietary resilience mechanisms: individuals with a strong cultural identity often advocate for traditional foods and maintain social connections through eating, strengthening their psychological resilience (Shatenstein et al., 2013).

Research by Taylor and Carr (2021) suggests that interventions aimed at strengthening resilience across all life stages have the potential to support successful ageing, with a significant proportion of older adults maintaining resilience primarily through social support and the adoption of adaptive mechanisms. Support from the community, family and professionals is crucial, as is access to care and available resources. Many older adults demonstrate resilience through social engagement, goal-directed behaviour and adaptive strategies (Carr et al., 2011). Southwick notes that resilience can be strengthened on multiple levels, including individual, family, community and cultural (Southwick et al., 2014).

A major motivation for successful adaptation and the development of resilient mechanisms is, undoubtedly, the desire to feel better and improve, or at least maintain, one's existing health status. James et al. (2022) report that participants in their study expressed a strong desire to feel better and explored the role of diet as a potential means of improving wellbeing. Through daily habits and ongoing engagement with the topic, healthy eating became a lifestyle for many participants. Experiencing the benefits of healthier eating and establishing firm values regarding diet and health supported the long-term maintenance of healthy eating. In this regard, self-care is another critical component of resilience strategies.

3.3.2 Dietary Resilience Strategies

According to Nygren (2005), the most frequently reported resilience strategies among older adults are social support, positive adaptation and the setting of personal goals. Older adults focus on the positive aspects of life, establish future-oriented goals and maintain hope for improvement. Setting personal goals provides structure and, when achieved, a sense of accomplishment. At the same time, pursuing these goals involves engaging in meaningful and fulfilling activities that give life purpose (Nygren et al., 2005).

The need to maintain motivation and social connections aligns with many conceptions of resilience and successful ageing that emphasise individual traits and behaviours (Rowe & Kahn, 1997). There is also a concept suggesting that resilience is a response to adversity (Hildon et al., 2010), and, according to Wiles et al. (2012), even individuals living with serious illness or health challenges can be considered resilient.

In this view, successful ageing is not limited to high levels of health or social connections; the potential of resilience lies in enabling people with disabilities to experience later life as meaningful and valuable, regardless of circumstances. This aligns with conceptualisations of resilience that emphasise balance, where resilience is not only about actively overcoming problems but also about accepting realities, such as disability or dependency (Reichstadt et al., 2010).

As people age and have fewer resources, social relationships can become a key source of resilience. Rowe and Kahn (1997) highlighted that social ties are essential for resilient ageing, and more recent studies confirm that support from family and community strengthens older adults' resilience, even in critical life situations (Wen et al., 2024). Antonucci et al. (2001) demonstrated how the quality of partnered relationships can impact depressive symptoms. Morelli et al. (2015) added that these relationships significantly improve psychological wellbeing and the ability to cope with adversity. Oswald et al. (2011), as well as the analysis by Duckworth et al. (2007), emphasise the positive influence of neighbourhood and broader community, with a sense of neighbourhood cohesion directly affecting the psychological resilience of older adults (Wang et al., 2019). While the objective quality of the environment plays a role, subjective perceptions of neighbourhood support appear to be a stronger predictor of life satisfaction than physical safety. Access to social networks, healthcare, transportation services and civic amenities is also increasingly crucial for the ability to age in place.

Orientation towards healthy eating is an important component of resilience mechanisms in older adults (Vesnaver & Keller, 2011). Learning and personal development are also significant, as they help keep the mind active and boost self-confidence, facilitating adaptation to changes in eating habits (Hayman et al., 2017). Self-care is another key element in the resilience strategies of older adults (Bolton et al., 2016).

Resilience mechanisms also include environmental mastery—creating a comfortable, safe and supportive environment that promotes independent living and enhances resilience (Nygren et al., 2005). Nyberg et al. (2018) report that participants in their study managed meals and eating habits by constantly adapting to new conditions arising from eating difficulties. They consciously planned what and when to eat, avoided certain foods and drinks and used simple tools, such as using both hands when drinking or relying solely on a spoon or fork, which help to manage the eating process while maintaining proper dining etiquette (Nyberg et al., 2018).

Gustaffson et al. (2003) note that the women studied had their own approaches to managing the situation, such as reorganising kitchen cabinets to reach everything they needed comfortably. They used special scissors to open milk cartons or cut food on the plate instead of using a knife. Some acquired a microwave to simplify heating food, whereas others bought an electric potato peeler. One strategy was shopping several times a week, purchasing smaller quantities each time, with smaller packages facilitating easier shopping. Some women modified their eating techniques to eat independently, for example, by switching to eating with a spoon or cutting all the food first and eating with one hand—methods easier on the wrist and usable when dining alone. When drinking, they could use a mug with a handle or hold it with both hands. Gustaffson also notes that older adults simplified food preparation by using pre-sliced bread, ready-made meatballs and canned meat sauces or soups. Setting the table was also simplified. Older adults who disliked eating alone often revitalised their social environment during meals with television, radio or even the presence of pets (Sidenvall et al., 2000).

Another resilience mechanism is a return to tradition. People actively create trajectories of food choices throughout their lives, which evolve dynamically while guiding future decisions (Sobal et al., 2014; Chong, 2022). For example, family meals and childhood food preferences form 'food roots', shaping food roles and eating identities that lead to lasting patterns. Returning to traditional foods and eating habits is a significant tool for many older adults to maintain personal and cultural identity. This dietary memory functions as a mechanism for recalling the past, strengthening the sense of belonging, continuity and temporal and spatial grounding (Wang et al., 2024). In the context of ageing, repeated rituals involving the preparation and consumption of traditional dishes can serve as a form of emotional resilience. Recalling family recipes, specific flavours or foods associated with particular life stages helps overcome feelings of loss or uncertainty. Food thus becomes not only a nutritional concern but also a means of preserving dignity, memory and self-determination (Wang et al., 2024). Jensen et al. (2019) point out that another area encountered in research, especially among women, was reconnecting with previous cooking skills. The composition and preparation of meals had been a key aspect of daily culinary practice for her respondents. Jensen's research demonstrates how previous and lifelong experiences with food and cooking become part of the strategies that give meaning to eating.

Sharing meals, or commensality, is another essential resilience strategy, especially for older adults living independently in their own homes. Eating is a significant social act that helps maintain relationships, a sense of belonging and identity (Vesnaver et al., 2012). For older adults, communal dining can be a key element of daily structure, a ritual that reduces loneliness and supports mental wellbeing. Vesnaver et al. (2012) show in their study that sharing meals can motivate older adults to adopt better eating habits and increase the enjoyment of food, which is particularly important for those at risk of malnutrition. The social aspects of eating are often more important than the actual content of the meal, and the presence of others can influence whether a person eats at all (Locher et al., 2005). Commensality is also linked to autonomy and dignity, as shared meals often allow older adults to actively participate in cooking, planning and sharing experiences. In the home environment, food thus becomes a tool for daily resilience and maintaining quality of life. De Castro (1994) found that caloric intake increases with the number of other people present at a meal. However, there are exceptions. For example, Sidenvall et al. (2000) found that older women reported a lack of appetite when eating with people they did not know.

The scientific literature increasingly emphasises the importance of pleasure and enjoyment of food as an important dietary resilience strategy. For some older adults, the enjoyment of food extends to food-related activities, such as meal planning, shopping and cooking (Vesnaver et al., 2012). Rappoport et al. (1993) found in their research that when explaining food choices, people almost always cited one or more of the following criteria: pleasure, health and availability. The idea that people commonly use these criteria to conceptualise their everyday eating behaviour is indirectly but substantially supported by several studies (Bailly et al., 2020), which show that even in childhood, people learn to categorise foods according to these criteria. According to Wang et al. (2024), the enjoyment of food is a primary source of health, wellbeing and meaning in life for older adults. Study results indicate that the experience of eating has a significant positive impact on their wellbeing and can bring a sense of happiness to older adults.

Closely related to the enjoyment of food is the concept of 'mindful eating'. The aim of mindful eating is to fully appreciate the process of acquiring, preparing and consuming food. Mindfulness focuses more on the process than the outcome, as control over food and the eating situation is crucial for developing dietary resilience (Vesnaver et al., 2016). Jensen et al. (2019) describe how older adults in Denmark develop meaningful eating strategies and explain that these strategies are related to the setting of eating habits, previous eating practices and body awareness. In research conducted by Nyberg et al. (2018), the ability to eat according to culturally accepted norms and maintain proper table manners was highly valued, representing an integral part of mindful eating. Vesnaver et al. (2012) report that individuals demonstrating dietary resilience emphasised the importance of mindful eating. They made conscious decisions about food and adjusted their eating to their financial resources, energy and time constraints. The connection between food, wellbeing and maintaining good health was pronounced.

Nelson (2017) explains the significance of mindful eating as an approach to food that focuses on sensory perception and the experience of eating. It has little to do with calories, carbohydrates, fats or proteins. The purpose of mindful eating is not weight loss, although those who adopt this eating style are likely to lose weight. The intention is to savour the moment and the food. It is no coincidence that within the mindful approach, people often choose to eat less, enjoy their food more and select foods aligned with their desired health benefits.

Learning and personal development is another resilience strategy. Resilient older adults continuously seek new information and acquire new skills in food selection and preparation. This helps them keep their minds active, boosts self-confidence and facilitates the acceptance of change (Hayman et al., 2017). Some older adults, as part of this resilience mechanism, show interest in cooking courses to learn more about grocery shopping and meal preparation techniques tailored to seniors with specific health conditions. They watch television, buy cooking magazines, visit online forums and share recipes and tips for healthy eating.

3.4 Conclusion

Dietary resilience in older adults results from the dynamic interplay of several interconnected factors. Individuals face physiological limitations, changes in life roles, social isolation and economic obstacles, yet many find ways to maintain appropriate eating habits, health and wellbeing. Key mechanisms include adaptive strategies such as meal planning, the use of practical aids, a flexible approach to eating and environmental mastery. Social and cultural dimensions—particularly support from family and community, a return to traditional foods and shared meals—contribute to the preservation of identity and a sense of belonging. Mindful eating and engagement in learning and new skills also play an important role by enhancing self-confidence and adaptability. Dietary resilience thus represents a complex mosaic of physical, psychological, social and cultural strategies aimed not only at maintaining nutrition and health but also at promoting autonomy, dignity and quality of life in older age. Successful ageing is both a matter of biological health and one's ability to actively manage change through interconnected adaptive mechanisms.

References

Ali-Kovero, K., Pietiläinen, O., Mauramo, E., Jäppinen, S., Rahkonen, O., Lallukka, T., & Kanerva, N. (2020). Changes in fruit, vegetable and fish consumption after statutory retirement: a prospective cohort study. British Journal of Nutrition, 123(12), 1390–1395. https://doi.org/10.1017/S0007114520000136

Andersen, S. S. (2021). The legacy of marriage: Using food to challenge traditional gender norms in widowhood. *Ageing & Society, 59*, Article 100966. https://doi.org/10.1016/j.jaging.2021.100966

Antonucci, T. C., Lansford, J. E., & Akiyama, H. (2001). Impact of Positive and Negative Aspects of Marital Relationships and Friendships on Well-Being of Older Adults. *Applied Developmental Science*, *5*(2), 68–75. https://doi.org/10.1207/S1532480XADS0502_2

Atchley RC. Retirement and leisure participation: continuity or crisis? Gerontologist. 1971 Spring;11(1):13–7. https://doi.org/10.1093/geront/11.1_Part_1.13. PMID: 5579223.

Bailey A, Bailey S, Bernoth M. 'I'd rather die happy': residents' experiences with food regulations, risk and food choice in residential aged care. A qualitative study. Contemp Nurse. 2017 Dec;53(6):597–606. https://doi.org/10.1080/10376178.2017.1361334. Epub 2017 Aug 9. PMID: 28758840.

Bailly N, Van Wymelbeke V, Maître I, Sulmont-Rossé C. The Assessment of Eating Pleasure among Older Adults: Development and Preliminary Validation of the Anticipatory and Consummatory Eating Pleasure (ACEPS). J Nutr Health Aging. 2020;24(6):606–613. https://doi.org/10.1007/s12603-020-1388-2. PMID: 32510113.

Blieszner, R., & Roberto, K. A. (2004). Friendship across the Life Span: Reciprocity in Individual and Relationship Development. In F. R. Lang & K. L. Fingerman (Eds.), *Growing together: Personal relationships across the lifespan* (pp. 159–182). Cambridge University Press.

Bolton, K. W., Praetorius, R. T., & Smith-Osborne, A. (2016). Resilience protective factors in an older adult population: A qualitative interpretive meta-synthesis. *Social Work Research, 40*(3), 171–182. https://doi.org/10.1093/swr/svw008

Bonanno, G. A. (2009). *The other side of sadness: What the new science of bereavement tells us about life after loss.* Basic Books/Hachette Book Group.

Calasanti, T., & King, N. (2005). Firming the Floppy Penis: Age, Class, and Gender Relations in the Lives of Old Men. *Men and Masculinities, 8*(1), 3–23. https://doi.org/10.1177/1097184X04268799

Carr, D. C., Komp, K. S., & Kunkel, S. R. (Eds.) (2011). *Gerontology in the era of the third age: New challenges and opportunities.* Springer Publishing.

Celidoni, M., Dal Bianco, C., Rebba, V., & Weber, G. (2020). Retirement and healthy eating. *Fiscal Studies, 41*(1), 199–219. https://doi.org/10.1111/1475-5890.12196

Chong MF. Dietary trajectories through the life course: opportunities and challenges. Br J Nutr. 2022 Jul 14;128(1):154–159. https://doi.org/10.1017/S0007114522001295. Epub 2022 Apr 27. PMID: 35475441.

Czech Statistical Office/Český statistický úřad (2025). https://csu.gov.cz/seniori-v-datech/predcasne-starobni-duchody?utm_source=chatgpt.com

de Castro JM. Family and friends produce greater social facilitation of food intake than other companions. Physiol Behav. 1994 Sep;56(3):445–5. https://doi.org/10.1016/0031-9384(94)90286-0. PMID: 7972393.

de Sire A, Ferrillo M, Lippi L, Agostini F, de Sire R, Ferrara PE, Raguso G, Riso S, Roccuzzo A, Ronconi G, Invernizzi M, Migliario M. Sarcopenic Dysphagia, Malnutrition, and Oral Frailty in Elderly: A Comprehensive Review. Nutrients. 2022 Feb 25;14(5):982. https://doi.org/10.3390/nu1405 0982. PMID: 35267957; PMCID: PMC8912303.

Delaney, M., & McCarthy, M. (2011). Food Choice and Health across the Life Course: A Qualitative Study Examining Food Choice in Older Irish Adults. *Journal of Food Products Marketing*, *17*(2–3), 114–140. https://doi-org.ezproxy.is.cuni.cz/https://doi.org/10.1080/10454446.2011.548717

Devine CM. A life course perspective: understanding food choices in time, social location, and history. J Nutr Educ Behav. 2005 May-Jun;37(3):121–8. https://doi.org/10.1016/s1499-4046(06)60266-2. PMID: 15904575.

Dondero KR, Falvey JR, Beamer BA, Addison O. Geriatric Vulnerabilities Among Obese Older Adults With and Without Sarcopenia: Findings From a Nationally Representative Cohort Study. J Geriatr Phys Ther. 2022 Jul-Sep 01;46(3):168–173. https://doi.org/10.1519/JPT.0000000000000358. Epub 2022 Aug 18. PMID: 35981333; PMCID: PMC9938079.

Duckworth AL, Peterson C, Matthews MD, Kelly DR. Grit: perseverance and passion for long-term goals. J Pers Soc Psychol. 2007 Jun;92(6):1087–101. https://doi.org/10.1037/0022-3514.92.6.1087. PMID: 17547490.

Elsner RJ. Changes in eating behavior during the aging process. Eat Behav. 2002 Spring;3(1):15–43. https://doi.org/10.1016/s1471-0153(01)00041-1. PMID: 15001018.

Govindaraju T, Owen AJ, McCaffrey TA. Past, present and future influences of diet among older adults - A scoping review. Ageing Res Rev. 2022 May;77:101600. https://doi.org/10.1016/j.arr.2022.101600. Epub 2022 Mar 4. PMID: 35248779.

Gustafsson K, Andersson I, Andersson J, Fjellström C, Sidenvall B. Older women's perceptions of independence versus dependence in food-related work. Public Health Nurs. 2003 May-Jun;20(3):237–47. https://doi.org/10.1046/j.0737-1209.2003.20311.x. PMID: 12716404.

Hayman, K. J., Kerse, N., & Consedine, N. S. (2017). Resilience in context: The special case of advanced age. *Aging & Mental Health, 21*(6), 577–585. https://doi.org/10.1080/13607863.2016.1196336

Hays, N. P., & Roberts, S. B. (2006). The anorexia of aging. *Physiology & Behavior, 88*(3), 257–266. https://doi.org/10.1016/j.physbeh.2006.05.029

Hildon Z, Montgomery SM, Blane D, Wiggins RD, Netuveli G. Examining resilience of quality of life in the face of health-related and psychosocial adversity at older ages: what is "right" about the way we age? Gerontologist. 2010 Feb;50(1):36–47. https://doi.org/10.1093/geront/gnp067. Epub 2009 Jun 23. PMID: 19549715.

Hoare, C. (2021). *The Oxford handbook of adult cognitive development*. Oxford University Press.

James A, Lawrence B, O'Connor M. Healthy Eating as a New Way of Life: A Qualitative Study of Successful Long-Term Diet Change. Inquiry. 2022 Jan-Dec;59:469580221090397. https://doi.org/10.1177/00469580221090397. PMID: 35418258; PMCID: PMC9016560.

Jensen T, Grønnow L, Jespersen AP. Eating strategies – a qualitative study of how frail, home-dwelling older people in Denmark develop strategies to form meaningful eating situations. *Ageing and Society*. 2019;39(3):590–608. https://doi.org/10.1017/S0144686X17001076

Jeppsson Grassman, E., & Whitaker, A. (2013). *Time, age and the failing body: A long life with disability*. In E. Jeppsson Grassman & A. Whitaker (Eds.), *Ageing with Disability: A Lifecourse Perspective* (pp. 17–34). Policy Press. https://doi.org/10.51952/9781447305231

Keller HH, Carrier N, Slaughter S, Lengyel C, Steele CM, Duizer L, Brown KS, Chaudhury H, Yoon MN, Duncan AM, Boscart VM, Heckman G, Villalon L. Making the Most of Mealtimes (M3): protocol of a multi-centre cross-sectional study of food intake and its determinants in older adults living in long term care homes. BMC Geriatr. 2017 Jan 13;17(1):15. https://doi.org/10.1186/s12877-016-0401-4. PMID: 28086754; PMCID: PMC5234152.

Kwon J, Suzuki T, Kumagai S, Shinkai S, Yukawa H. Risk factors for dietary variety decline among Japanese elderly in a rural community: a 8-year follow-up study from TMIG-LISA. Eur J Clin Nutr. 2006 Mar;60(3):305–11. https://doi.org/10.1038/sj.ejcn.1602314. PMID: 16234831.

Lagström H, Lahdenperä M, Ravyse C, Akbaraly T, Kivimaki M, Pentti J, Stenholm S, Head J. Changes in food habits during the transition to retirement: the Whitehall II cohort study. J Epidemiol Community Health. 2025 Jan 13;79(2):131–137. https://doi.org/10.1136/jech-2024-222690. PMID: 39353723; PMCID: PMC11874461.

Lange-Chenier H. Older Canadians at risk of undernourishment. CMAJ. 2013 Jul 9;185(10):E473. https://doi.org/10.1503/cmaj.109-4482. Epub 2013 May 27. PMID: 23713069; PMCID: PMC3708025.

Leahy, A. (2023) "Disability Identity in Older Age? - Exploring Social Processes that Influence Disability Identification with Ageing", *Disability Studies Quarterly* 42(3–4). https://doi.org/10.18061/dsq.v42i3-4.7780
Liu W, Galik E, Boltz M, Nahm ES, Resnick B. Optimizing Eating Performance for Older Adults With Dementia Living in Long-term Care: A Systematic Review. Worldviews Evid Based Nurs. 2015 Aug;12(4):228–35. https://doi.org/10.1111/wvn.12100. Epub 2015 Jun 29. PMID: 26122316.
Locher JL, Ritchie CS, Roth DL, Baker PS, Bodner EV, Allman RM. Social isolation, support, and capital and nutritional risk in an older sample: ethnic and gender differences. Soc Sci Med. 2005 Feb;60(4):747–61. https://doi.org/10.1016/j.socscimed.2004.06.023. PMID: 15571893; PMCID: PMC2763304.
Morales F, Montserrat-de la Paz S, Leon MJ, Rivero-Pino F. Effects of Malnutrition on the Immune System and Infection and the Role of Nutritional Strategies Regarding Improvements in Children's Health Status: A Literature Review. Nutrients. 2023 Dec 19;16(1):1. https://doi.org/10.3390/nu16010001. PMID: 38201831; PMCID: PMC10780435.
Morelli SA, Lee IA, Arnn ME, Zaki J. Emotional and instrumental support provision interact to predict well-being. Emotion. 2015 Aug;15(4):484–93. https://doi.org/10.1037/emo0000084. Epub 2015 Jun 22. PMID: 26098734; PMCID: PMC4516598.
Nelson JB. Mindful Eating: The Art of Presence While You Eat. Diabetes Spectr. 2017 Aug;30(3):171–174. https://doi.org/10.2337/ds17-0015. PMID: 28848310; PMCID: PMC5556586.
Neri CM, D'Alba L. Nutrition and Healthy Aging: Prevention and Treatment of Gastrointestinal Diseases. Nutrients. 2021 Nov 30;13(12):4337. https://doi.org/10.3390/nu13124337. PMID: 34959889; PMCID: PMC8706789.
Nyberg M, Olsson V, Örtman G, Pajalic Z, Andersson HS, Blücher A, Lindborg, Wendin K, Westergren A. The meal as a performance: food and meal practices beyond health and nutrition. Ageing & Society. 2018;38(1):83–107 https://doi.org/10.1017/S0144686X16000945
Nygren, B., Aléx, L., Jonsén, E., Gustafson, Y., Norberg, A., & Lundman, B. (2005). Resilience, sense of coherence, purpose in life and self-transcendence in relation to perceived physical and mental health among the oldest old. *Aging & Mental Health, 9*(4), 354–362. https://doi.org/10.1080/1360500114415
Ogg, J., & Renaut, S. (2019). The influence of family and professional life-course histories on economic activity among older French workers. *Ageing & Society, 39*(10), 2242–2266. https://doi.org/10.1017/S0144686X18001459

Oswald F, Jopp D, Rott C, Wahl HW. Is aging in place a resource for or risk to life satisfaction? Gerontologist. 2011 Apr;51(2):238–50. https://doi.org/10.1093/geront/gnq096. Epub 2010 Nov 19. PMID: 21097552.

Park JH, Kang SW. Nutritional Risk, Depression, and Physical Function in Older People Living Alone. Healthcare (Basel). 2024 Jan 10;12(2):164. https://doi.org/10.3390/healthcare12020164. PMID: 38255052; PMCID: PMC10815494.

Patriota, P., Marques-Vidal, P. (2021). Retirement is associated with a decrease in dietary quality. *Clinical Nutrition ESPEN, 45*, 206–212. https://doi.org/10.1016/j.clnesp.2021.07.004

Payette H, Coulombe C, Boutier V, Gray-Donald K. Nutrition risk factors for institutionalization in a free-living functionally dependent elderly population. J Clin Epidemiol. 2000 Jun;53(6):579–87. https://doi.org/10.1016/s0895-4356(99)00186-9. PMID: 10880776.

Payette H, Shatenstein B. Determinants of healthy eating in community-dwelling elderly people. Can J Public Health. 2005 Jul-Aug;96 Suppl 3:S27–31, S30–5. English, French. PMID: 16042161.

Phinney A, Chaudhury H, O'Connor DL. Doing as much as I can do: the meaning of activity for people with dementia. Aging Ment Health. 2007 Jul;11(4):384–93. https://doi.org/10.1080/13607860601086470. PMID: 17612802.

Plastow NA, Atwal A, Gilhooly M. Food activities and identity maintenance in old age: a systematic review and meta-synthesis. Aging Ment Health. 2015;19(8):667–78. https://doi.org/10.1080/13607863.2014.971707. Epub 2014 Nov 6. PMID: 25373998; PMCID: PMC4440631.

Quandt, S. A., Arcury, T. A., & Bell, R. A. (1998). Self-management of nutritional risk among older adults: A conceptual model and case studies from rural communities. *Journal of Aging Studies, 13*(4), 351–368. https://doi.org/10.1016/S0890-4065(98)90027-X

Rappoport L, Peters GR, Downey R, McCann T, Huff-Corzine L. Gender and age differences in food cognition. Appetite. 1993 Feb;20(1):33–52. https://doi.org/10.1006/appe.1993.1004. PMID: 8452376.

Reichstadt J, Sengupta G, Depp CA, Palinkas LA, Jeste DV. Older adults' perspectives on successful aging: qualitative interviews. Am J Geriatr Psychiatry. 2010 Jul;18(7):567–75. https://doi.org/10.1097/jgp.0b013e3181e040bb. PMID: 20593536; PMCID: PMC3593659.

Roderka MN, Puri S, Batsis JA. Addressing Obesity to Promote Healthy Aging. Clin Geriatr Med. 2020 Nov;36(4):631–643. https://doi.org/10.1016/j.cger.2020.06.006. Epub 2020 Aug 16. PMID: 33010899; PMCID: PMC7533351.

Rowe JW, Kahn RL. Successful aging. Gerontologist. 1997 Aug;37(4):433–40. https://doi.org/10.1093/geront/37.4.433. PMID: 9279031.

Sakurai R, Kawai H, Suzuki H, Kim H, Watanabe Y, Hirano H, Ihara K, Obuchi S, Fujiwara Y. Association of Eating Alone With Depression Among Older Adults Living Alone: Role of Poor Social Networks. J Epidemiol. 2021 Apr 5;31(4):297–300. https://doi.org/10.2188/jea.JE20190217. Epub 2020 Apr 18. PMID: 32307350; PMCID: PMC7940972.

Sarafrazi N, Wambogo EA, Shepherd JA. Osteoporosis or low bone mass in older adults: United States, 2017–2018. NCHS Data Brief, no 405. Hyattsville, MD: National Center for Health Statistics. 2021. https://doi.org/10.15620/cdc:103477external icon

Schiffman SS. Influence of medications on taste and smell. World J Otorhinolaryngol Head Neck Surg. 2018 Mar 26;4(1):84–91. https://doi.org/10.1016/j.wjorl.2018.02.005. PMID: 30035266; PMCID: PMC6051304.

Shahar DR, Schultz R, Shahar A, Wing RR. The effect of widowhood on weight change, dietary intake, and eating behavior in the elderly population. J Aging Health. 2001 May;13(2):189–99. https://doi.org/10.1177/089826430101300202. PMID: 11787511.

Shatenstein, B., Gauvin, L., Keller, H. *et al.* Baseline determinants of global diet quality in older men and women from the NuAge cohort. *J Nutr Health Aging* 17, 419–425 (2013). https://doi.org/10.1007/s12603-012-0436-y

Sidenvall, B., Nydahl, M., & Fjellström, C. (2000). The Meal as a Gift—The Meaning of Cooking Among Retired Women. *Journal of Applied Gerontology, 19*(4), 405–423. https://doi.org/10.1177/073346480001900403

Sobal, J., Bisogni, C.A., & Jastran, M. (2014). Food Choice Is Multifaceted, Contextual, Dynamic, Multilevel, Integrated, and Diverse. *Mind, Brain, and Education, 8*, 6–12.

Southwick SM, Bonanno GA, Masten AS, Panter-Brick C, Yehuda R. Resilience definitions, theory, and challenges: interdisciplinary perspectives. Eur J Psychotraumatol. 2014 Oct 1;5. https://doi.org/10.3402/ejpt.v5.25338. PMID: 25317257; PMCID: PMC4185134.

Stahl ST, Schulz R. Changes in routine health behaviors following late-life bereavement: a systematic review. J Behav Med. 2014 Aug;37(4):736–55. https://doi.org/10.1007/s10865-013-9524-7. Epub 2013 Jul 24. PMID: 23881308; PMCID: PMC4197803.

Sydner Y. Mattsson, C. Fjellström, M. Lumbers, B. Sidenvall & M. Raats. (2007). *Food Habits and Foodwork*, Food, Culture & Society, 10:3, 367–387, https://doi.org/10.2752/155280107X239845

Taylor MG, Carr D. Psychological Resilience and Health Among Older Adults: A Comparison of Personal Resources. J Gerontol B Psychol Sci Soc Sci. 2021 Jun 14;76(6):1241–1250. https://doi.org/10.1093/geronb/gbaa116. PMID: 32750146.

Vesnaver E, Keller HH, Payette H, Shatenstein B. Dietary resilience as described by older community-dwelling adults from the NuAge study "if there is a will -there is a way!". Appetite. 2012 Apr;58(2):730–8. https://doi.org/10.1016/j.appet.2011.12.008. Epub 2011 Dec 16. PMID: 22200412.

Vesnaver E, Keller HH, Sutherland O, Maitland SB, Locher JL. Alone at the Table: Food Behavior and the Loss of Commensality in Widowhood. J Gerontol B Psychol Sci Soc Sci. 2016 Nov;71(6):1059–1069. https://doi.org/10.1093/geronb/gbv103. Epub 2015 Nov 10. PMID: 26556790; PMCID: PMC6083990.

Vesnaver E, Keller HH. Social influences and eating behavior in later life: a review. J Nutr Gerontol Geriatr. 2011;30(1):2–23. https://doi.org/10.1080/01639366.2011.545038. PMID: 23286638.

Wacka E, Nicikowski J, Jarmuzek P, Zembron-Lacny A. Anemia and Its Connections to Inflammation in Older Adults: A Review. J Clin Med. 2024 Apr 2;13(7):2049. https://doi.org/10.3390/jcm13072049. PMID: 38610814; PMCID: PMC11012269.

Wang X, Qi J, Zhang K, Xie H, Wu X. The joy of eating: how eating experiences enhance the well-being of older adults. Front Public Health. 2024 Sep 9;12:1438964. https://doi.org/10.3389/fpubh.2024.1438964. PMID: 39314795; PMCID: PMC11417023.

Wang, R., Chen, H., Liu, Y., Lu, Y., & Yao, Y. (2019). Neighborhood social reciprocity and mental health among older adults in China: the mediating effects of physical activity, social interaction, and volunteering. *BMC Public Health*, *19*(1), Article 1036. https://doi.org/10.1186/s12889-019-7385-x

Wen, Z., Wang, H., Liang, Q., Liu, L., Zhang, W., & Zhang, X. (2024). Mediating effect of social support and resilience between loneliness and depression in older adults: A systematic review and meta-analytic structural equation modeling. *Journal of Affective Disorders, 365*, 246–257. https://doi.org/10.1016/j.jad.2024.08.062

Westergren A., Hagell P., Sjödahl Hammarlund C. (2014). *Malnutrition and risk of falling among elderly without home-help service — A cross sectional study*. The Journal of nutrition, health and aging, Volume 18, Issue 10, 2014, Pp. 905–911, ISSN 1279-7707, https://doi.org/10.1007/s12603-014-0469-5.

Whitelock E. & Ensaff H. (2018). *On Your Own: Older Adults' Food Choice and Dietary Habits.* Nutrients 2018, 10, 413; https://doi.org/10.3390/nu10040413

Wiles JL, Wild K, Kerse N, Allen RES. Resilience from the point of view of older people: 'There's still life beyond a funny knee'. Soc Sci Med. 2012 Feb;74(3):416–424. https://doi.org/10.1016/j.socscimed.2011.11.005. Epub 2011 Dec 14. PMID: 22204841.

Williams K. The transition to widowhood and the social regulation of health: consequences for health and health risk behavior. J Gerontol B Psychol Sci Soc Sci. 2004 Nov;59(6):S343-9. https://doi.org/10.1093/geronb/59.6.s343. PMID: 15576865.

Wills, W., & Dickinson, A. (2023). Vulnerability to Food Insecurity among Older People: The Role of Social Capital. *Sociological Research Online*, *28*(4), 946–963. https://doi.org/10.1177/13607804231170516

World Health Organization. (2018). *Ageing and health.* WHO. https://doi.org/10.1016/S0140-6736(15)60217-5

Zhang M, Zhang N, Zhou M, Ma G. Association between neighborhood food environment and dietary diversity score among older people in Beijing, China: A cross-sectional study. Front Nutr. 2022 Sep 20;9:903214. https://doi.org/10.3389/fnut.2022.903214. PMID: 36211503; PMCID: PMC9534378.

4

Gender and Dietary Resilience in Later Life

Abstract This chapter examines the role of gender in shaping the eating practices and dietary resilience of older adults. Eating is conceptualised not merely as a biological necessity but as a culturally and gender-conditioned activity that intersects with identity, autonomy and social roles. Women tend to exhibit healthier dietary patterns, reflecting their lifelong caregiving responsibilities, greater health literacy and broader social networks. These experiences enable women to respond flexibly to age-related changes, developing strategies that support resilience despite structural inequalities and economic constraints. Men, by contrast, often relate to food through affirmations of masculinity, autonomy and physical strength. Life transitions such as the loss of traditional household roles may disrupt men's eating routines but can also foster new forms of resilience, including engagement with cooking, modern food technologies and active decision-making in food choices. Both men and women employ adaptive strategies, yet these are deeply influenced by socially constructed gender norms, which shape the meanings attached to food, body image and health. Overall, gendered dynamics reveal that food is a medium through which older adults negotiate resilience, social belonging and the maintenance of identity.

E. Ferrarová, *Dietary Resilience Strategies in Older Adults with Physical Disabilities*,
https://doi.org/10.1007/978-3-032-22186-5_4

Keywords Gender · Dietary patterns · Resilience · Body image

4.1 Introduction

This chapter examines the ways in which gender influences and shapes dietary behaviours and resilience strategies among older adults. It focuses on how lifelong gender norms affect eating patterns in later life, and how these patterns either persist or change with age. By exploring the gender-specific dynamics of eating, the chapter aims to shed light on the adaptive and resilience strategies employed by men and women.

Gender differences in the diets of older adults are well documented and reflect a combination of biological, cultural and psychosocial factors. Older women often display healthier dietary patterns than men, with higher consumption of fruits, vegetables, whole grains and water. In contrast, men tend to prefer fattier foods, meat and fast food, and they consume alcoholic beverages more frequently (Warren, 2024). These differences are shaped not only by individual preferences but also by social norms and cultural expectations related to gender. Studies have shown that women tend to eat more regularly, place greater emphasis on healthy eating and are more motivated to take care of their health. Men, on the other hand, more often seek foods high in fat and with strong flavour and are motivated more by the pleasure of eating than by its nutritional value. Such behavioural differences can influence food choices, energy intake, overall health in later life and the development of resilience mechanisms (Sobal et al., 2014; Lombardo et al., 2024).

In relation to health in old age, gender also plays an important role. Women generally demonstrate higher levels of health literacy regarding nutrition and are more likely to seek information about healthy eating, read food labels, consult their dietary habits with physicians and actively participate in preventive programmes. This enables them to better understand their own nutritional needs and adjust their behaviour accordingly, for example, in connection with chronic illnesses. This pronounced motivation among women to care for their health provides them with tools to act more purposefully and strategically in the domain of nutrition compared to men (von Bothmer & Fridlund, 2005).

Everyday food-related decision-making, shaped by gender norms, also influences how older adults perceive their own bodies (Furnham et al., 2002; Gross et al., 2005; Gorini et al., 2025). While among younger adults these differences are often linked to pressures related to bodily ideals, in older adults, gender-specific patterns are reflected more in the relationship to the body as a source of identity, health and control (Clarke & Korotchenko, 2011).

Older women often face a dual burden: on the one hand, the physical changes associated with ageing, and on the other, cultural norms that continue to value thinness and self-control as markers of female identity. Qualitative research highlights that, especially among older women, perceptions of health, thinness and body size play an important role in dietary habits and preferences (Jensen et al., 2019; Gustafsson & Sidenvall, 2002). This is also reflected in eating behaviours, where women more often than men show dietary restrictions, feelings of guilt when eating and efforts to control food intake, even when they are no longer exposed to such strong social control as in earlier stages of life (Holmes et al., 2023). At the same time, however, according to Tunaley (1999), some older women adopt an indifferent attitude towards body size and food, thereby rejecting societal pressures associated with the (appropriate) body image.

Older men, too, face their own specific challenges related to food. The existence of gendered patterns of perception and behaviour—and their importance in how older adults understand their dietary situations—is confirmed by an American study focusing on frail men and how their relationship to cooking influences their eating habits. The study found that men in general, and widowers in particular, associate food with physical strength and perceive it as a means of maintaining the body and control over their lives (Moss et al., 2007).

The findings show that gender influences not only how older adults eat, but also how they understand their bodies, health and social roles through food. Such patterns can be seen as part of broader resilience strategies. For women, dietary restriction or health-oriented behaviour can serve as a way to maintain control and identity in old age, whereas, for men, cooking and eating may become a means of preserving independence and strength.

4.2 Gendered Dietary Patterns in Later Life

The significance of food and eating in later life from a gender perspective, particularly for individuals with certain limitations in everyday functioning, holds an important place in gerontological research.

4.2.1 Feeding the Family

The study of the relationship between gender and food can help to understand the context in which the relationship of women and men to food takes place (Avakian & Haber, 2005). The home is often a place of work for women, consisting largely of activities connected with 'feeding'. Food-related activities are simultaneously physical, mental and social, and they are what create the family. For example, when choosing food, a woman must decide according to the wishes of other family members and the local conception of what counts as 'proper' food (DeVault, 1991). DeVault maintains that this work of feeding is invisible as work and, although central to the construction of family, women themselves often deny that it is work. In relationships between women and men, food functions as a tool of power. Scholars agree that in no society do women have more power than men; nevertheless, lively debates continue over whether food work and its distribution give women power within the family or merely confirm their subordinate role (Allen & Sachs, 2007). Most feminist scholars strictly maintain that the domestic sphere reproduces patriarchal values and women's physical, intellectual and ideological subordination. Although women generally bear responsibility for their role, it is men who set the rules and control their fulfilment (Gouws, 2024). Moreover, family food is 'men's food', because it is determined by men's dietary preferences (Sobal, 2005). Foodwork is also strongly gendered: women plan menus more often than men, do the shopping and cook. This is connected with the concept of man as the breadwinner. Yet, women tend to cook 'men's food'. When men cook, it is often a hypermasculine performance of meat preparation. Masculine cooking frequently occurs outdoors and over fire (Sobal, 2005).

A gender perspective can also be applied to the eating patterns of older adults, which serve as a basis for the development of resilience strategies. In terms of everyday roles, one important contribution in this area is the study by Jensen et al. (2019). A key finding of her research is that men tend to perceive food primarily as a means of maintaining control over their lives—that is, as a tool of power. Several of Jensen's respondents described feeling they had control over themselves in food-related situations, even though the actual food work or procurement was carried out by women, such as their daughters or domestic helpers.

Through a gendered lens, the position of widowed individuals is particularly interesting. Davidson et al. (2009) point out that a widowed person must adapt to a new role and tasks previously performed by their spouse. Among older generations, where the division of household duties, including those related to food, is often strongly gendered, widowers may find themselves for the first time in life in a situation where they have to prepare food on their own. Similarly, widows may suddenly face a new situation in which they cook only for themselves and according to their own tastes (Sidenvall et al., 2000). While women often perceive liberation from domestic responsibilities as a positive aspect, most widowers report feeling less free after taking on these responsibilities (Davidson et al., 2009). Vesnaver (2011) qualitatively examined how older widows managed their eating behaviour independently. She found that some women realised that many of their eating habits had been shaped by their husbands' preferences and, subsequently, adjusted their routines to better reflect their own tastes. Others, however, felt disoriented without the duty of care, and food lost its meaning for them. For these women, the significance of cooking was closely tied to the role of preparing meals for the family and husband, and in the absence of someone to cook for, meal preparation lost its purpose.

For men not previously accustomed to cooking or planning meals, the loss of a partner is often a turning point, and their eating habits may deteriorate. They often develop a one-sided or irregular diet (Vesnaver et al., 2016), whereas, according to Davidson et al. (2009), for older men who have always lived alone, meal preparation is part of their masculine identity and serves both to express it and to confirm its continuity. At times, meal preparation can challenge masculine identity, as it represents a role traditionally held by women (Davidson et al., 2009). Interestingly, when men apply principles of efficiency and technical skill in describing meal preparation, they frame this activity as similar to paid work, thereby elevating its status from a domestic duty (perceived as feminine) to specialised work (perceived as masculine) (Cusack, 2017).

4.2.2 Gender Differences in Food Choices

Most experts agree that the gendering of food is a cultural rather than a biological construct (Allen & Sachs, 2007). Foods are gendered in different ways across cultures and historical periods. In post-industrial Western societies like ours, 'men's foods' typically include meat (preferably beef), hamburgers, potatoes and beer, while 'women's foods' include salads, pasta, yoghurt, fruit and chocolate (Leiserowitz et al., 2020). According to Sobal (2005), gender in food can be studied through singular or multiple models of gendering. Singular models of masculinity typify foods as either masculine or feminine, with men and women 'doing gender' by consuming gender-appropriate foods. Meat, and especially red meat, represents the archetypal masculine food. Contemporary Western notions of 'proper meals' are centred around meat and form the basis of couple meals, reproducing broader patterns of male dominance.

Independence is a hallmark of contemporary Western masculinity. To 'eat like a man' often means refusing to give up foods discouraged by authorities. In this way, men frequently perform masculinity through food—by eating what they want rather than what they are supposed to eat (Sobal, 2005).

These gender stereotypes are also reflected in the eating practices of older adults, where older men consume more meat than older women. However, when crossing the barrier of age 65, there may be an inverse correlation between masculinity and ageing (Ritzel & Mann, 2021).

By contrast, today's women often minimise or avoid meat consumption, thereby resisting or demystifying masculine meat eating. Whereas masculinity is demonstrated by what men eat, femininity is usually demonstrated by what women do not eat. Men often view meat as 'too heavy, too strong' for women, and indeed, food taboos restricting meat consumption are more commonly applied to women than to men. These stereotypes persist into older age as well. Older women tend to eat less meat and more fish, fruit and vegetables, which also reflects their relationship to their health (Dean et al., 2009).

Dietary patterns of older adults are also gendered in terms of their relationship to health. In general, women engage in health-promoting behaviours much more than men and have healthier lifestyles (Vesnaver & Keller, 2011; Plastow et al., 2015). Some men also want to eat healthily and reduce their consumption of red meat while increasing their intake of vegetables, specifically in connection with ageing (Sobal, 2005). Healthier dietary patterns are more often observed among people with higher education (Sobal, 2005).

Quandt et al. (1998) concluded in their research that older women are at higher nutritional risk than men. From a biological perspective, women have specific nutritional needs related to the menstrual cycle, pregnancy, breastfeeding and menopause. These stages increase the requirements for iron, calcium, folate and other micronutrients, and their deficiency can more easily lead to malnutrition (Wells et al., 2020). The risk of insufficient food intake and loss of appetite increases more often in older women than in men because older women live alone, have lower incomes and face greater social isolation as a result of widowhood (Locher et al., 2005). In older women, frailty syndrome also occurs more frequently, which is closely associated with malnutrition (Gobbens et al., 2010). As a result of these factors, the risk of undernutrition in older women may be up to twice as high as in men of the same age, especially in those living alone or in institutional care (de van der Schueren et al., 2020).

Older women eat more healthily than men, but although health theoretically holds a dominant position, its principles often struggle with the strong social influence of entrenched eating habits. From a gender perspective, it is interesting that this tension between health recommendations and subjective experience applies to both women and men. It often appears as a symbolic expression of agency: choosing certain foods against the advice of healthcare professionals serves as an act of identity affirmation and an exercise of control over the present (Freire Paz et al., 2025).

4.2.3 Sociocultural Dimensions of Gendered Diets

The social dimension of eating is important because shared meals or participation in community dining programmes help maintain social independence and prevent loneliness. For men, eating among others can motivate continued interest in cooking and regular food intake (Hughes et al., 2004). Older men generally have less active social networks than women, which limits their opportunities to share meals or seek help (Locher et al., 2005; Cornwell and Waite, 2009). This limited social contact can reduce opportunities for meal sharing and emotional support, leading to poorer dietary quality (Locher et al., 2005). Women participate more frequently than men in communal meals or social activities involving food, which promotes appetite and increases food intake (Vesnaver et al., 2012).

Psychological factors also play a significant role in the eating behaviours of older women and men. Eating disorders such as anorexia and bulimia primarily affect women, which is linked to societal pressure towards thinness and the ideal female body (Bordo, 1993; Halliwell & Dittmar, 2003). Additionally, women more often experience depression and anxiety, which can affect both their appetite and overall relationship with food. Dietary behaviours aimed at controlling body weight can lead to chronic deficiencies in essential nutrients.

Geographic and cultural factors can further exacerbate malnutrition among women. In some regions of the world, women have limited access to food, particularly where food distribution within the household prioritises men and children (FAO, 2023). Older women, often living alone, are especially at risk due to the loss of social contact, reduced motivation to prepare meals and physical difficulties with shopping and cooking. Economic inequality between genders also affects diet quality, as women tend to have lower food security (FAO, 2023).

Dietary patterns in later life are strongly gendered. Older women more frequently choose healthier food practices but are simultaneously more vulnerable to malnutrition due to widowhood, social isolation or lower incomes. Men, on the other hand, tend to prefer meals higher in meat and fat, and, after losing a partner, they often experience a decline in eating habits, although some perceive cooking as part of their identity.

These differences, however, are not merely a reproduction of traditional roles—they also create space for resilience strategies: women can reinforce control and identity through healthier eating or meal restrictions, while men may seek new forms of autonomy and continuity with their life story through food preparation.

4.3 Dietary Resilience Strategies by Gender

Older adults strive to maintain independence in later life through food and related activities in ways that encompass practical, symbolic and psychological aspects. Just as there are differences in dietary patterns between men and women, there are also gendered differences in the adoption of dietary resilience strategies. Men and women employ different approaches to coping with stress and declining health, which are influenced by social, cultural and biological factors. There are various levels of dietary resilience strategies, and all are gendered.

For many older adults, meal preparation is a key daily activity that allows them to maintain a sense of autonomy and manage everyday life. For women in particular, cooking holds a strong significance as part of their identity and domestic role, making the preservation of this ability important for dignity and maintaining routine (Locher et al., 2005; Vesnaver et al., 2012). Regular cooking itself can easily be considered a form of resilience. Even more, older women demonstrate resilience by adapting to age-related limitations through modifying recipes to suit their abilities and adjusting the kitchen environment to facilitate independent meal preparation (Dean et al., 2009). Conversely, men often use aids in later life, such as ergonomic utensils, pre-prepared meals, delivery services or technologies that help them maintain self-sufficiency in eating and meal preparation without complete dependence on others (Parsons et al., 2019).

Women are considered more resilient because they have better skills in home meal preparation, cook more frequently than men, plan meals and manage food efficiently. These are skills acquired over a lifetime in the traditionally female role of household caregiver (Vesnaver & Keller,

2011). Women can also rely on stronger social networks as they maintain social ties more effectively, enabling them to share meals, obtain help with shopping or cooking and preserve the social aspect of eating (Mehranfar et al., 2025). Women are more likely to adopt new dietary habits (e.g., due to illness) and adapt more easily to changes without losing interest in food (Grzywacz et al., 2012). Results from Gustafsson and Sidenvall (2002) show that women in later life adopted various methods of coping with their situations and created their own strategies to manage life despite declining health.

Planning and decision-making around food also represent a way to maintain control over one's body, health and daily routine, thereby developing resilience strategies. Women are more actively engaged in learning about healthy nutrition and adapt their diets according to health needs, maintaining an active role in managing their health (Dean et al., 2009). Daily shopping, cooking and eating routines provide psychological support for stability and a sense of normalcy. The loss of these routine activities is often associated with a loss of meaning and identity (Locher et al., 2005).

Many of the challenges women face in later life are related to cumulative gender inequalities shaped over the life course, including economic insecurity, caregiving responsibilities, health burdens and complex structural constraints (UN Women, 2021; Meliou & Mallett, 2021). Societal expectations that primarily place long-term responsibility for caring for children, older adults or the sick on women can result in significant limitations to career and income growth, which in later life manifest as economic insecurity and a reduced ability to secure adequate nutrition (Meliou & Mallett, 2021). Research from the World Health Organization (WHO) has shown that older women more often experience multiple chronic conditions, higher levels of functional limitations and lower financial security than men of the same age, with these disparities deepening when women live alone or are socioeconomically marginalised (WHO, 2020).

Nevertheless, there is evidence that women demonstrate higher levels of resilience than men in nutrition and eating. This resilience consists particularly in their ability to adapt to demanding life situations and changing conditions (D'Amico et al., 2020). This ability is not biologically predetermined but is shaped by lifelong social, cultural and economic factors. Women are traditionally responsible for organising household food, and, especially during times of crisis or scarcity, they are the ones who plan purchases, prepare meals, make decisions about priorities and often place the needs of children, partners or elderly relatives above their own. Although this role often comes without social recognition, it can contribute to developing the ability to respond quickly and flexibly to nutritional challenges. These behavioural strategies can be understood as a form of nutritional resilience, serving as immediate coping methods and long-term health strategies (Darmon & Drewnowski, 2015).

Women's nutritional resilience is inextricably linked to gender roles that often assign them responsibility for caring for others. While societal expectations contribute to the development of specific skills and strategies in women, they also imply increased physical, psychological and time burdens. Female resilience in nutrition can thus be interpreted as a means of survival under structurally unequal conditions rather than as a mark of privilege (DeVault, 1991). Even this resilience, however, is not inexhaustible. Women from low-income households, single mothers or members of marginalised groups face numerous barriers that significantly weaken their adaptive capacity. A lack of financial resources, time constraints or limited access to quality food and healthcare can lead to the deterioration of their nutritional status. Long-term stress, caregiving responsibilities and societal pressure to ensure the 'proper' functioning of the household may result in older women facing health and nutritional problems they have spent their lives trying to prevent (Popay et al., 2021). Kinsel (2005) notes that among the factors identified as key to resilience in his research sample of women were social connectedness and internal resources, with curiosity and openness towards others playing a crucial role in their lives. Continuing life despite adverse events and engaging in unconventional or nontraditional behaviour supported the preservation of their identity.

One of the key resilience strategies is sharing food, especially among women. This can include communal meals or cooking for others, particularly for family. Sidenvall et al. (2000) explain this by noting that women were traditionally responsible for preparing, cooking and serving food in private households; for older generations of women, this duty was common. One reason may be that cooking is closely tied to female identity and rationality. For example, Oleschuk (2019) shows that home cooking is still perceived as a gendered organisation of daily eating, where women assume both emotional and practical responsibility for family meals. Mazzonetto studied three generations of women and their relationship to cooking for others. Only the youngest generation considered cooking a personal choice; the middle and oldest generations considered it their duty, which could also provide a sense of usefulness (Mazzonetto et al., 2025). According to Arganini et al. (2012), women value eating with friends and relatives more than men. Similarly, Sidenvall et al. (2000) found that newly widowed women reported a loss of motivation to cook after their husband's death. When living alone, cooking loses its purpose. These experiences of losing a partner illustrate how deeply gender roles are embedded in the everyday practice of food. These differences also extend to the broader dietary patterns of men and women. According to a 2022 Gallup survey, nearly three-quarters of women (76%) reported enjoying cooking, compared to 40% of men. The pleasure derived from preparing and consuming food is thus a vital resilience strategy.

In their empirical study, Jensen et al. (2019) report that the men developed resilience through positive experiences with food and the sense that they were able to obtain or even prepare meals. To achieve this, they mobilised their strength despite physical weakness or illness. However, they also note that, in some cases, these strategies could lead to the rejection of the foods most nutritionally appropriate for them. Moss et al. (2007) also mention the mobilisation of physical strength as a resilience strategy in men. The results of their empirical study showed that men in their sample tended to perceive food and life in two contrasting ways: some spoke at a more concrete level, emphasising the need to eat in order to exist and to live, whereas others discussed food as a symbol of life's pleasures. According to Davidson (2004), there are significant differences in the social dimensions of eating between men living alone and married men. Most men living alone eat outside the home, which provides opportunities for social interaction, choice and the satisfaction of being able to pay for their own meals—all symbolising their presence in the world. Older men often tend to downplay their performance of traditionally 'female' food preparation skills, emphasising the continuity of their sense of masculinity, asserting their independence, control over their lives and strength. Despite the losses of old age, older men often experience personal resilience in having survived and learned new ways to adapt to their increasingly limited world (Davidson, 2004).

Nutritional resilience strategies in older age take many forms, from practical adaptive measures and maintaining daily routines to symbolic and social aspects associated with cooking and sharing meals. Women tend to display greater flexibility and adaptability, reflecting their lifelong experience with household food responsibility and broader social networks. However, this resilience is often accompanied by increased burden and structural inequalities that limit their options. Empirical studies indicate that men develop dietary resilience in later life through the mobilisation of physical strength and positive experiences with food, which reinforce their sense of autonomy, masculinity and control over life, even though these strategies may sometimes lead to the rejection of nutritionally appropriate foods.

4.4 Body Image, Gender and Diet

Despite the changes accompanying older age, older adults often demonstrate remarkable adaptability and resilience, finding ways to maintain a positive body image and quality of life through various adaptive strategies, including those related to eating (Jensen et al., 2019; Nyberg et al., 2018).

The relationship between the body, gender, age, food and health is complex and influenced by a wide range of factors, including genetics, hormones, lifestyle, cultural norms and socioeconomic status (Delaney & McCarthy, 2014; Host et al., 2016). One's relationship with their own body, which significantly affects eating behaviour, is strongly gendered. Body size carries diverse and often contrasting meanings for older women and men, shaped by social ideals of beauty, gender identity and age. Both women and men may experience pressure to maintain a certain appearance throughout their lives, but specific ideals of attractiveness change with age. While youthfulness and thinness are often prioritised in younger individuals, older adults may be considered attractive for other qualities, such as wisdom, maturity or self-confidence. Nevertheless, gendered expectations regarding appearance can persist, with women more frequently subjected to scrutiny and pressure to maintain a youthful appearance than men (Halliwell & Dittmar, 2003). Many older women express dissatisfaction with their physical appearance, reflecting the intergenerational influence of the 'thin ideal' (Bordo, 1993). According to Counihan (1999), women's dissatisfaction with their body weight and shape in Western societies reflects their historically subordinate social position (Counihan, 1999).

Tunaley et al. (1999) found that the differing relationships men and women have with their bodies are the result of deeply ingrained social expectations that dictate what is considered a desirable body and how women and men should relate to food and eating. At the same time, some women adopt a laissez-faire attitude towards body size and eating, rejecting pressures pertaining to weight and food. This approach is linked to their perception of this stage of life as a period of freedom and to the belief in the inevitability of weight gain with age. Gendered eating patterns significantly influence changes in body size and weight over time. For women, these patterns are often associated with caloric restriction and plant-based fats, whereas for men, weight loss is primarily linked to the consumption of animal proteins (Rein et al., 2024).

Older men may experience various bodily changes with age, such as muscle loss, increased body fat, reduced skin elasticity and postural changes. These changes affect how men perceive their bodies, especially in comparison to their younger selves or to societal ideals of masculinity (Calasanti and King, 2005). Some older men may feel pressure to conform to traditional masculine ideals emphasising strength, muscularity and physical appearance (Adams and Taylor, 2015). These bodily experiences are also closely tied to the social roles men occupy throughout life. Roles such as 'family provider' or physically strong worker can reinforce the perception of the body as a tool for performance and social value. When older men leave the workforce or can no longer fulfil these expected roles, their relationship with their body may shift—from seeing it as a source of strength and productivity to viewing it through the lens of health, vulnerability and the need for care.

These factors also influence men's relationship with food, often perceived more as a routine in older age. Men typically view eating as a habitual, routine activity that provides their bodies with necessary energy. Although they are aware of healthy eating principles, they often exhibit scepticism or are resistant to nutritional guidance, and they may perceive healthy eating as monotonous and unsatisfying.

While many considerations of the body in older age still relate to ideals of beauty and social expectations, the focus does gradually shift towards health. Emphasising health may overlap with the ongoing effort to maintain a certain appearance, but it can also offer an alternative perspective in which the body is valued more for its functionality and vitality than for its aesthetic qualities (Grenier & Hanley, 2007; Gustafsson & Sidenvall, 2002). Research indicates that older women tend to eat less than men and prefer foods that support weight control. For example, Waren (2024) identified differences in food preferences, with women more often choosing vegetables, whole grains and healthier options compared to men.

Thus, the significance of body image in older age is not only a matter of individual aesthetics but is also connected to how men and women adapt their eating strategies to their changing bodies and social expectations, becoming an integral part of their resilience strategies.

4.5 Conclusion

Gender significantly shapes the daily food practices of older adults as well as the ways in which they maintain and develop resilience in later life. This chapter focused primarily on the idea that eating is not merely a biological necessity but also a culturally and gender-conditioned activity. Women more often than men exhibit healthier eating patterns, which relates to their lifelong role as caregivers; higher health literacy; and broader social networks. This experience enables them to respond more flexibly to age-related changes and limitations, creating strategies that support their nutritional resilience. On the other hand, they also bear the burden of structural inequalities and economic insecurity, often limiting their options.

Men face different challenges. Their relationship with food is frequently more closely tied to affirming masculine identity, autonomy and physical strength. Especially after widowhood or the loss of traditional role divisions, men may find themselves in situations that threaten the quality of their diet. However, these circumstances also present opportunities for new forms of resilience by cooking, using modern technologies or excersing agency in food choices. These gendered dynamics demonstrate that food is not merely a matter of nutrition but also a medium through which identity, resilience and social belonging are negotiated.

References

Adams, R. G., and Taylor, E. M. 2015. Friendship and Happiness in the Third Age, in Demir M. (ed), Friendship and Happiness: Across the Life-Span and in Different Cultures, Dordrecht: Springer. https://doi.org/10.1007/978-94-017-9603-3

Allen, P., C. Sachs. 2007. Women and Food Chains: The Gendered Politics of Food. *The International Journal of Sociology of Agriculture and Food* 15(1): 1–23. https://doi.org/10.48416/ijsaf.v15i1.42

Arganini, C., Saba, A., Comitato, R., Virgili, F., & Turrini, A. (2012). Gender Differences in Food Choice and Dietary Intake in Modern Western Societies. InTech. https://doi.org/10.5772/37886

Avakian, A. V., B. Haber (eds.). 2005. *From Betty Crocker to Feminist Food Studies: Critical Perspectives on Women and Food.* Amherst: University of Massachusetts Press.

Baker L, Gringart E. Body image and self-esteem in older adulthood. *Ageing and Society.* 2009;29(6):977-995. https://doi.org/10.1017/S0144686X09008721

Bordo, Susan, 1993. Unbearable Weight : Feminism, Western Culture, and the Body. Berkeley :University of California Press.

Calasanti, T., & King, N. (2005). Firming the Floppy Penis: Age, Class, and Gender Relations in the Lives of Old Men. *Men and Masculinities*, *8*(1), 3-23. https://doi.org/10.1177/1097184X04268799 (Original work published 2005)

Cederholm T, Jensen GL, Correia MITD, Gonzalez MC, Fukushima R, Higashiguchi T, Baptista G, Barazzoni R, Blaauw R, Coats AJS, Crivelli AN, Evans DC, Gramlich L, Fuchs-Tarlovsky V, Keller H, Llido L, Malone A, Mogensen KM, Morley JE, Muscaritoli M, Nyulasi I, Pirlich M, Pisprasert V, de van der Schueren MAE, Siltharm S, Singer P, Tappenden K, Velasco N, Waitzberg D, Yamwong P, Yu J, Van Gossum A, Compher C; GLIM Core Leadership Committee, GLIM Working Group. GLIM criteria for the diagnosis of malnutrition - A consensus report from the global clinical nutrition community. J Cachexia Sarcopenia Muscle. 2019 Feb;10(1):207–217. https://doi.org/10.1002/jcsm.12383. PMID: 30920778; PMCID: PMC6438340.

Clarke LH, Korotchenko A. Aging and the Body: A Review. Can J Aging. 2011 Sep 1;30(3):495-510. https://doi.org/10.1017/S0714980811000274. PMID: 24976674; PMCID: PMC4072651.

Cornwell EY, Waite LJ. Social disconnectedness, perceived isolation, and health among older adults. J Health Soc Behav. 2009 Mar;50(1):31-48. https://doi.org/10.1177/002214650905000103. PMID: 19413133; PMCID: PMC2756979.

Counihan, C.M. (1999). The Anthropology of Food and Body: Gender, Meaning and Power (1st ed.). Routledge. https://doi.org/10.4324/9781315656540

Cusack, I. (2017). Food, masculinities, and home. interdisciplinary perspectives. *Food, Culture & Society*, *21*(1), 121–123. https://doi-org.ezproxy.is.cuni.cz/https://doi.org/10.1080/15528014.2017.1406281

D'Amico D, Parrott MD, Greenwood CE, Ferland G, Gaudreau P, Belleville S, Laurin D, Anderson ND, Kergoat MJ, Morais JA, Presse N, Fiocco AJ. Sex differences in the relationship between dietary pattern adherence and cognitive function among older adults: findings from the NuAge study. Nutr J. 2020 Jun 20;19(1):58. https://doi.org/10.1186/s12937-020-00575-3. PMID: 32563260; PMCID: PMC7306140.

Darmon N, Drewnowski A. Contribution of food prices and diet cost to socioeconomic disparities in diet quality and health: a systematic review and analysis. Nutr Rev. 2015 Oct;73(10):643–60. https://doi.org/10.1093/nutrit/nuv027. Epub 2015 Aug 25. PMID: 26307238; PMCID: PMC4586446.

Davidson K., S. Arber, H. Marshall, Gender and food in later life: shifting roles and relationships, Editor(s): Monique Raats, Lisette de Groot, Wija van Staveren, In Woodhead Publishing Series in Food Science, Technology and Nutrition, Food for the Ageing Population, Woodhead Publishing, 2009, Pages 110–127, ISBN 9781845691936, https://doi.org/10.1533/9781845695484.1.110.

Davidson, K. (2004). "Why Can't a Man Be More like a Woman?": Marital Status and Social Networking of Older Men. *The Journal of Men's Studies, 13*(1), 25-43. https://doi.org/10.3149/jms.1301.25 (Original work published 2004)

de van der Schueren MAE, Keller H; GLIM Consortium; Cederholm T, Barazzoni R, Compher C, Correia MITD, Gonzalez MC, Jager-Wittenaar H, Pirlich M, Steiber A, Waitzberg D, Jensen GL. Global Leadership Initiative on Malnutrition (GLIM): Guidance on validation of the operational criteria for the diagnosis of protein-energy malnutrition in adults. Clin Nutr. 2020 Sep;39(9):2872–2880. https://doi.org/10.1016/j.clnu.2019.12.022. Epub 2020 Jun 11. PMID: 32563597.

Dean M, Raats MM, Grunert KG, Lumbers M; Food in Later Life Team. Factors influencing eating a varied diet in old age. Public Health Nutr. 2009 Dec;12(12):2421–7. https://doi.org/10.1017/S1368980009005448. Epub 2009 Apr 6. PMID: 19344544.

Delaney M, McCarthy MB. Saints, sinners and non-believers: the moral space of food. A qualitative exploration of beliefs and perspectives on healthy eating of Irish adults aged 50–70. Appetite. 2014 Feb;73:105–13. https://doi.org/10.1016/j.appet.2013.10.017. Epub 2013 Oct 31. PMID: 24184539.

DeVault M. 1991. Feeding the family. University of Chicago Press.

FAO. (2023). *The State of Food Security and Nutrition in the World 2023: Urbanization, agrifood systems transformation and healthy diets across the rural–urban continuum.* Food and Agriculture Organization of the United Nations. https://doi.org/10.4060/cc3017en

Freire Paz E, Rivero Jiménez B, Caballero DC, Mariano Juárez L. Loneliness, Food Practices, and Ageing: The Inclusion of Qualitative Evidence in Health Promotion Programmes. Nutrients. 2025 Sep 8;17(17):2906. https://doi.org/10.3390/nu17172906. PMID: 40944294; PMCID: PMC12430704.

Furnham A, Badmin N, Sneade I. Body image dissatisfaction: gender differences in eating attitudes, self-esteem, and reasons for exercise. J Psychol. 2002 Nov;136(6):581-96. https://doi.org/10.1080/00223980209604820. PMID: 12523447.

Gallup. (2022) Wellbeing Through Cooking Global Insights Into Cooking Enjoyment and Eating Together. file:///D:/Gallup-Ajinomoto%20Group-Wellbeing%20Through%20Cooking-Report.pdf

Gobbens RJ, Luijkx KG, Wijnen-Sponselee MT, Schols JM. Toward a conceptual definition of frail community dwelling older people. Nurs Outlook. 2010 Mar-Apr;58(2):76–86. https://doi.org/10.1016/j.outlook.2009.09.005. PMID: 20362776.

Gorini S, Camajani E, Cava E, Feraco A, Armani A, Amoah I, Filardi T, Wu X, Strollo R, Caprio M, Padua E, Lombardo M. Gender differences in eating habits and sports preferences across age groups: a cross-sectional study. J Transl Med. 2025 Mar 12;23(1):312. https://doi.org/10.1186/s12967-025-06311-x. PMID: 40075461; PMCID: PMC11900493.

Gouws, A. (2024). The State, the Domestic Sphere and Patriarchy: Thinking with Belinda Bozzoli. *Agenda, 38*(1), 53–62. https://doi-org.ezproxy.is.cuni.cz/https://doi.org/10.1080/10130950.2025.2466640

Grenier, A., & Hanley, J. (2007). Older Women and 'Frailty': Aged, Gendered and Embodied Resistance. *Current Sociology, 55*(2), 211-228. https://doi.org/10.1177/0011392107073303 (Original work published 2007)

Gross SM, Gary TL, Browne DC, LaVeist TA. Gender differences in body image and health perceptions among graduating seniors from a historically black college. J Natl Med Assoc. 2005 Dec;97(12):1608–19. PMID: 16396053; PMCID: PMC2640720.

Grzywacz JG, Stoller EP, Brewer-Lowry AN, Bell RA, Quandt SA, Arcury TA. Gender and health lifestyle: an in-depth exploration of self-care activities in later life. Health Educ Behav. 2012 Jun;39(3):332–40. https://doi.org/10.1177/1090198111405195. Epub 2011 Jun 1. PMID: 21632439; PMCID: PMC3693089.

Gustafsson K, Sidenvall B. Food-related health perceptions and food habits among older women. J Adv Nurs. 2002 Jul;39(2):164-73. https://doi.org/10.1046/j.1365-2648.2002.02256.x. PMID: 12100660.

Halliwell, E., & Dittmar, H. (2003). A Qualitative Investigation of Women's and Men's Body Image Concerns and Their Attitudes Toward Aging. *Sex Roles: A Journal of Research, 49*(11-12), 675–684. https://doi.org/10.1023/B:SERS.0000003137.71080.97

Holmes BA, Roberts CL. Diet quality and the influence of social and physical factors on food consumption and nutrient intake in materially deprived older people. Eur J Clin Nutr. 2011 Apr;65(4):538-45. https://doi.org/10.1038/ejcn.2010.293. Epub 2011 Jan 26. PMID: 21266981.

Host, Alison; McMahon, Anne T.; Walton, Karen L.; and Charlton, Karen E., “Factors influencing food choice for independently living older people - a systematic literature review” (2016). Faculty of Science, Medicine and Health - Papers: part A. 3693. https://ro.uow.edu.au/smhpapers/3693

Hughes G, Bennett KM, Hetherington MM. Old and alone: barriers to healthy eating in older men living on their own. Appetite. 2004 Dec;43(3):269-76. https://doi.org/10.1016/j.appet.2004.06.002. PMID: 15527929.

Jensen T, Grønnow L, Jespersen AP. Eating strategies – a qualitative study of how frail, home-dwelling older people in Denmark develop strategies to form meaningful eating situations. *Ageing and Society*. 2019;39(3):590-608. https://doi.org/10.1017/S0144686X17001076

Kinsel B. Resilience as adaptation in older women. J Women Aging. 2005;17(3):23-39. https://doi.org/10.1300/J074v17n03_03. PMID: 16186093.

Leiserowitz, A.; Ballew, M.; Lacroix, K.; Marlon, J.; Talaty, U. (2020). Exploring Gender Differences in the American Diet. New Haven, CT: Yale Program on Climate Change Communication.

Locher JL, Ritchie CS, Roth DL, Baker PS, Bodner EV, Allman RM. Social isolation, support, and capital and nutritional risk in an older sample: ethnic and gender differences. Soc Sci Med. 2005 Feb;60(4):747-61. https://doi.org/10.1016/j.socscimed.2004.06.023. PMID: 15571893; PMCID: PMC2763304.

Lombardo M, Feraco A, Armani A, Camajani E, Gorini S, Strollo R, Padua E, Caprio M, Bellia A. Gender differences in body composition, dietary patterns, and physical activity: insights from a cross-sectional study. Front Nutr. 2024 Jul 11;11:1414217. https://doi.org/10.3389/fnut.2024.1414217. PMID: 39055386; PMCID: PMC11271261.

Mazzonetto AC, Melo JNM, Dean M, Fiates GMR. From ‘cooking wife’ to ‘cooking mother’: Exploring generational shifts in perceptions regarding domestic cooking practices. Nutr Diet. 2025 Feb;82(1):115-122. https://doi.org/10.1111/1747-0080.12910. Epub 2024 Oct 25. PMID: 39450578.

Mehranfar S, Ceolin G, Madani Civi R, Keller H, Murphy RA, Cohen TR, Conklin AI. Gender, Adverse Changes in Social Engagement and Risk of Unhealthy Eating: A Prospective Cohort Study of the Canadian Longitudinal Study on Aging (2011-2021). Nutrients. 2025 Mar 13;17(6):1005. https://doi.org/10.3390/nu17061005. PMID: 40290021; PMCID: PMC11946033.

Meliou, E., & Mallett, O. (2021). Negotiating Gendered Ageing: Intersectional Reflexivity and Experiences of Incongruity of Self-Employed Older

Women. *Work, Employment and Society, 36*(1), 101-118. https://doi.org/10.1177/0950017021994489 (Original work published 2022)
Moss, Sidney Z., Miriam S. Moss, Janet E. Kilbride, and Robert L. Rubinstein. 2007. 'Frail Men's Perspectives on Food and Eating'. Journal of Aging Studies 21(4):314–24. https://doi.org/10.1016/j.jaging.2007.05.006.
Nyberg M, Olsson V, Örtman G, et al. The meal as a performance: food and meal practices beyond health and nutrition. *Ageing and Society.* 2018;38(1):83-107. https://doi.org/10.1017/S0144686X16000945
Oleschuk, M. (2019). Gender, Cultural Schemas, and Learning to Cook. *Gender & Society, 33*(4), 607-628. https://doi.org/10.1177/0891243219839669 (Original work published 2019)
Parsons TJ, Papachristou E, Atkins JL, Papacosta O, Ash S, Lennon LT, Whincup PH, Ramsay SE, Wannamethee SG. Physical frailty in older men: prospective associations with diet quality and patterns. Age Ageing. 2019 May 1;48(3):355-360. https://doi.org/10.1093/ageing/afy216. PMID: 30668624; PMCID: PMC6503938.
Plastow NA, Atwal A, Gilhooly M. Food activities and identity maintenance in old age: a systematic review and meta-synthesis. Aging Ment Health. 2015;19(8):667–78. https://doi.org/10.1080/13607863.2014.971707. Epub 2014 Nov 6. PMID: 25373998; PMCID: PMC4440631.
Popay J, Whitehead M, Ponsford R, Egan M, Mead R. Power, control, communities and health inequalities I: theories, concepts and analytical frameworks. Health Promot Int. 2021 Oct 13;36(5):1253-1263. https://doi.org/10.1093/heapro/daaa133. PMID: 33382890; PMCID: PMC8515177.
Quandt, S. A., Arcury, T. A., & Bell, R. A. (1998). Self-management of nutritional risk among older adults: A conceptual model and case studies from rural communities. *Journal of Aging Studies, 13*(4), 351–368. https://doi.org/10.1016/S0890-4065(98)90027-X.
Rein M, Elkan M, Godneva A, Dolev NC, Segal E. Sex-specific dietary habits and their association with weight change in healthy adults. BMC Med. 2024 Nov 6;22(1):512. https://doi.org/10.1186/s12916-024-03730-3. PMID: 39501340; PMCID: PMC11539530.
Ritzel C, Mann S. The Old Man and the Meat: On Gender Differences in Meat Consumption across Stages of Human Life. Foods. 2021 Nov 15;10(11):2809. https://doi.org/10.3390/foods10112809. PMID: 34829090; PMCID: PMC8619336.
Sidenvall, B., Nydahl, M., & Fjellström, C. (2000). The Meal as a Gift—The Meaning of Cooking Among Retired Women. *Journal of Applied Gerontology, 19*(4), 405-423. https://doi.org/10.1177/073346480001900403

Sobal, J. (2005). Men, meat, and marriage: models of masculinity. *Food and Foodways, 13*(1–2), 135–158. https://doi-org.ezproxy.is.cuni.cz/https://doi.org/10.1080/07409710590915409

Sobal, J., Bisogni, C.A., & Jastran, M. (2014). Food Choice Is Multifaceted, Contextual, Dynamic, Multilevel, Integrated, and Diverse. *Mind, Brain, and Education, 8*, 6-12.

Tunaley JR, Walsh S, Nicolson P. 'I'm not bad for my age': the meaning of body size and eating in the lives of older women. *Ageing and Society*. 1999;19(6):741-759. https://doi.org/10.1017/S0144686X99007515

UN Women (2021): The impact of COVID-19 on older women: Insights and recommendations. https://www.unwomen.org/en/digital-library/publications/2021/03/the-impact-of-covid-19-on-older-women

Vesnaver E, Keller HH, Payette H, Shatenstein B. Dietary resilience as described by older community-dwelling adults from the NuAge study "if there is a will -there is a way!". Appetite. 2012 Apr;58(2):730-8. https://doi.org/10.1016/j.appet.2011.12.008. Epub 2011 Dec 16. PMID: 22200412.

Vesnaver E, Keller HH, Sutherland O, Maitland SB, Locher JL. Alone at the Table: Food Behavior and the Loss of Commensality in Widowhood. J Gerontol B Psychol Sci Soc Sci. 2016 Nov;71(6):1059–1069. https://doi.org/10.1093/geronb/gbv103. Epub 2015 Nov 10. PMID: 26556790; PMCID: PMC6083990.

Vesnaver, E., & Keller, H. H. (2011). Social Influences and Eating Behavior in Later Life: A Review. *Journal of Nutrition in Gerontology and Geriatrics, 30*(1), 2–23. https://doi-org.ezproxy.is.cuni.cz/https://doi.org/10.1080/01639366.2011.545038

von Bothmer MI, Fridlund B. Gender differences in health habits and in motivation for a healthy lifestyle among Swedish university students. Nurs Health Sci. 2005 Jun;7(2):107-18. https://doi.org/10.1111/j.1442-2018.2005.00227.x. PMID: 15877687.

Warren A (2024) The relationship between gender differences in dietary habits, neuroinflammation, and Alzheimer's disease. *Front. Aging Neurosci.* 16:1395825. https://doi.org/10.3389/fnagi.2024.1395825

Wells JC, Sawaya AL, Wibaek R, Mwangome M, Poullas MS, Yajnik CS, Demaio A. The double burden of malnutrition: aetiological pathways and consequences for health. Lancet. 2020 Jan 4;395(10217):75–88. https://doi.org/10.1016/S0140-6736(19)32472-9. Epub 2019 Dec 15. PMID: 31852605; PMCID: PMC7613491.

World Health Organization (2020). Decade of healthy ageing: Baseline report. https://doi.org/10.4060/cb1507en

5

Qualitative Study on Dietary Resilience in Later Life

Abstract This chapter explores the concept of dietary resilience in older adults. It presents findings from a qualitative study focused on everyday eating practices and strategies that enable the maintenance of independence, health and quality of life in later life. The analysis of twenty-three participant interviews revealed several key dimensions of resilience: independence in eating, gendered culinary and caregiving practices, mindful eating and the enjoyment of food, adaptation to health limitations, diversification of food sources, the use of social networks and knowledge of healthy eating principles. The results show that resilience is not limited to functional adaptations such as modifying recipes or using kitchen aids but also encompasses emotional, social and cultural dimensions ranging from sensory enjoyment and the preservation of traditions to engagement in social relationships and community activities. The study emphasises that dietary resilience results from the interplay between personal motivation, culturally learned practices and available material and social resources.

Keywords Dietary resilience · Ageing · Independence · Gender · Mindful eating · Enjoyment of eating

E. Ferrarová, *Dietary Resilience Strategies in Older Adults with Physical Disabilities*,
https://doi.org/10.1007/978-3-032-22186-5_5

5.1 Introduction

This chapter presents a qualitative study aimed at understanding how older adults living in their own households respond to age- and health-related limitations and how they develop strategies of dietary resilience. The chapter first outlines the research aims and methodology, then introduces the participants and ethical considerations. The following sections present the main findings, their interpretation in the discussion and, finally, a summary of the most important insights.

5.1.1 Research Aims

Older adults face many changes that come with ageing. They must respond and adapt to new life circumstances, including those related to age- and health-related disadvantages, whether physical or mental. This research focuses on how older people, who continue to live at home, respond to these changes and what strategies and mechanisms of dietary resilience they develop to cope with new situations.

The study concentrated on food selection, meal planning, shopping, cooking, perceptions of food and commensality, and sharing meals with friends and family, as well as other food-related activities. It addresses food intake, as this represents one of the most important—if not the most essential—components in the daily activities of older adults and is key to meeting their nutritional, psychological and social needs.

The specific aims of the qualitative research were (a) to identify the dietary resilience strategies used by older adults living in their own households and (b) to explore and describe the key forms of dietary resilience in relation to gender.

The research questions were as follows:

1. What dietary resilience strategies do older adults living in their own households used to adapt to changing life circumstances?
2. How do gender differences manifest themselves in the dietary resilience strategies of older adults living at home?

5.1.2 Methodology

In order to answer the research questions, a qualitative ethnographic approach was adopted that allowed for the in-depth exploration of older adults' experiences and practices related to food and eating. The present qualitative study is part of a broader project, 'Meanings of Food Intake in Old Age', which explores the subjective significance of food and eating practices in the context of life changes in later life.

A multi-method ethnographic approach was implemented, combining semi-structured in-depth interviews and participant observation. This enabled the researchers to gain insight into the dietary habits of twenty-three older adults (aged 65+), living in their own homes, either alone or with others, in various Czech cities. The participants were recruited through the personal and professional networks of the research team, as well as through senior organisations. After a verbal agreement, they were contacted by phone and informed in detail about the study. All participants signed an informed consent form, which included the information that they could withdraw from the research at any time.

An interview guide covered key themes, including menu planning, food sourcing, preparation, eating, festive meals, self-provisioning, food sharing, body image and eating with physical limitations. Interviews were audio recorded, transcribed verbatim and analysed using Atlas.ti. A conventional content analysis was used, capturing both manifest and latent meanings. This was important in order to uncover the factors involved in how older men and women perceived and performed their food and eating practices in everyday life. Singular codes were then identified, and codes with similar content were organised into different categories. Observation notes were carefully read and analysed in the same way as the interview material. The observations helped to capture the meal's performative aspects and facilitated an understanding of the participants' eating patterns. The combination of interviews and participant observation allowed for methodological triangulation, strengthening the validity of the findings by capturing both articulated narratives and observed practices.

5.1.3 Participants

The selection criteria for participants were set at age 65+ and living in their own homes. The sampling was deliberately structured to achieve a balanced representation of women and men. Participants were selected within the researchers' social networks and included individuals with similar socioeconomic backgrounds. The sample thus ensured that the study would be conducted among participants living in comparable conditions.

A total of twenty-three individuals[1] (12F and 11M) aged 65–92 participated in the study; all lived in their own homes alone or with a partner. Participants were recruited from major cities: Prague, Brno and Ostrava, as well as their suburban areas.

In terms of education, seven participants had a university degree (4F and 3M), ten had completed secondary education with a school-leaving certificate (7F and 3M), five had vocational training (1F and 4M) and one woman had only an elementary education.

With respect to marital status, ten participants were married (4F and 6M), nine were widowed (7F and 2M), two were divorced (1F and 1M) and two were separated (2M). Nineteen participants were fully retired (10F and 7 M), while four remained professionally active after retirement (2F and 4M).

Participants provided a subjective assessment of their socioeconomic status (SES) on a scale of 1–10 (1 = very good, 10 = very bad) (Table 5.1).

The participants' subjective assessments of their economic situation were mostly in the lower range of the scale (1–5), indicating an overall rather positive perception of their socioeconomic status. The most frequently selected score was 1 (very good; 6 participants), with women choosing this option more often than men. Only two participants (both women) reported poorer ratings, in the range of 7–8. The average rating was 3.8 for women and 3.3 for men, showing a slightly more positive perception of SES among men.

[1] F = female; M = male, Mar = married; W = widow, widower; S = separated; D = divorced.

Table 5.1 Subjective assessment of socioeconomic status (SES)

Score (1–10)	Women	Men	Total
1	4	2	6
2	1	2	3
3	1	2	3
4	1	1	2
5	2	2	4
6	0	0	0
7	1	1	2
8	2	0	2
Not assessed	–	1	1
Total	12	11	23
Average	3.8	3.3	3.6

Information on health status was obtained through interviews, in which some participants explicitly or implicitly described their health issues, as well as through a questionnaire that included a section on health, including a subjective self-assessment of health (Table 5.2). Participants rated their health on a scale from 1 to 10 (1 = very good, 10 = very poor) as follows:

Participants' subjective assessments of their health status varied considerably. Most respondents were clustered around the mid-range of the scale (4–7), indicating that they perceived their health as satisfactory, though with certain difficulties. Only a small number of participants (4

Table 5.2 Subjective assessment of health status

Score (1–10)	Women	Men	Total
1	2	0	2
2	2	0	2
3	2	1	3
4	2	2	4
5	1	1	2
6	1	1	2
7	1	2	3
8	0	3	3
9	1	0	1
Not assessed	0	1	1
Total	12	11	23
Average	3.9	6	4.9

women) rated their health as very good (1–2), whereas higher scores (8–9) appeared at the opposite end of the spectrum and were reported more often by men. Overall, women tended to perceive their health somewhat more positively than men, although for both genders, the majority of ratings were mid-range rather than at the top of the scale.

Most participants had more than one diagnosis: 14 had musculoskeletal disorders, 8 had cardiovascular diseases, 8 had diabetes, 8 suffered from digestive system disorders, 2 had high blood pressure, 2 were obese and 4 reported dental problems. Many participants experienced multiple health limitations simultaneously. Thirteen participants (7F + 6M) reported being restricted in performing daily activities, while ten (5F + 5M) did not feel restricted. Four participants (2F + 2M) required assistance from others, whereas nineteen (11F + 8M) did not need help.[2]

When comparing the participants' subjective assessments of their economic situation and health, both dimensions predominantly fell within the mid-range of the scales. While most participants perceived their economic situation relatively positively (with an average score around 3–4), their health assessments were more dispersed and tended towards less favourable values (4–7). This suggests that a good or acceptable SES does not necessarily correspond to a positive perception of one's own health. An interesting finding is the gender difference: women rated their economic situation slightly lower than men, yet their health evaluations were overall more positive. This contrast highlights the complex relationship between socioeconomic status and health, showing that the subjective experience of ageing is shaped not only by economic conditions but also by culture and gender.

From a resilience perspective, this difference is significant, as it demonstrates that even when participants face health limitations or economic disadvantage, they find ways to compensate—for example, through adapting dietary practices, sharing meals or using social relationships as

[2] If a participant's disability was not reported in either the interview or the questionnaire and was only observed or inferred by the anthropologist conducting the interview, this observation was recorded in the field journal but was not included in the analysis of data obtained from the interviews.

supportive resources. Resilience, therefore, is reflected not only in objective indicators of health or finances but especially in older adults' ability to maintain a sense of stability and meaningfulness in daily life despite deteriorating conditions.

These findings on subjectively perceived economic situation and health provide an important context for further analysis. They show that even when participants face various forms of disadvantage, their everyday strategies and ways of coping with changes reflect a certain degree of resilience. In Sect. 5.2. 'Findings', these adaptive mechanisms will be illustrated in more detail in the context of dietary practices.

5.1.4 Data Collection

All of the team members participated in conducting interviews and observations, asking questions, recording answers, taking notes and photographing whenever possible. In four interviews, the participant's partner also took part, providing additional contextual information. The interviews were conducted in participants' homes (14), in a café (2), at the university where they attended the University of the Third Age (U3A) (4), at the seniors organisation Život 90 (2) and at the workplace (1). Each session lasted between 45 and 120 minutes. The interviews took place between September 2023 and December 2023.

An interview guide was used to facilitate the interviews, ensuring that all main topics were covered. The guide included several themes and subquestions covering different aspects of food and meal practices: menu planning, food sourcing/shopping, food preparation, eating, related activities, fine dining, dining out, weight/body issues, self-provisioning and related activities. The interview began by asking the participant to describe his or her usual daily meal structure, and the subsequent course of the interview depended on the response to this open-ended question. All interviews were audio-recorded and transcribed verbatim. With the participants' consent, photographs of their kitchens, refrigerators, pantries and set tables were taken and included as part of the data.

5.1.5 Data Analysis

Interviews were coded using a deductive content analysis, guided by pre-defined categories derived from the theoretical framework on dietary resilience and gender (Elo & Kyngäs, 2008). This approach allowed us to systematically capture instances of pre-conceptualised phenomena, while remaining open to emerging nuances.

The recorded interviews were transcribed verbatim and uploaded into the software Atlas.ti, allowing us to code them using our established codes. Code evaluation was carried out by all team members who were familiar with the complete data sets (transcripts, field notes and records) from specific households. The interviews were coded using conventional (latent and manifest) content analysis to highlight the text's apparent and deeper or latent meanings. This was important for uncovering factors involved in how older men and women perceive and perform their food and meal practices in everyday life. Singular codes were then identified, and codes with similar content were organised into different categories. The notes taken from the observations were thoroughly read and analysed in the same way as the interview material.

In the subsequent phase, a discursive approach (Seymour-Smith, 2015) was employed to examine how gender performativity was expressed in participants' eating practices and mealtime interactions. While the primary coding followed a deductive content analysis, this discursive lens enabled a more nuanced interpretation of how gendered behaviours and meanings manifested within the pre-defined categories. The observational material was then used to triangulate and validate the interview findings, capturing the performative aspects of mealtime practices.

5.1.6 Ethical Considerations

In accordance with the ethical standards put forward in the 1964 Declaration of Helsinki and its later amendments, and in accordance with the Directive No. 5/2015 'Research Ethics at Masaryk University', the participants were informed orally and in writing of the purpose of the study both before and at the time of the interviews. Each participant signed an informed consent form for video and audio recording and data processing. Participation was voluntary, and participants were informed of their right to discontinue participation at any point. All information was treated confidentially. The participants' personal data and information were encrypted and anonymised. Each participant was assigned a number and a different name to ensure consistency in the anonymisation.

Each team member signed the Researcher's Code of Conduct. In accordance with the ethical standards laid out in the 1964 Declaration of Helsinki, its later amendments, and Masaryk University's Directive No. 5/2015, the project obtained approval from the school's Ethics Committee for Research (EKV MU). The management and administration of the project activities worked to respect the balance between work and family life and support age and gender equality.

In accordance with the General Data Protection Regulation (EU 2016/679; GDPR), the data controller is Masaryk University, Žerotínovo nám. 617/9, 601 77 Brno. The contact of the data protection officer is poverenec@muni.cz and ekv@muni.cz.

The Ethics Committee of Masaryk University (EKV MU) is registered with the Office for Human Research Protections (OHRP)—U.S. Department of Health and Human Services, within the OHRP Database for Registered IORGs and IRBs under the following identifiers: Institutional review board (IRB) organization (IORG) registration Number: IORG0010793 IRB Number: IRB00012800 Masaryk University IRB #1.

5.2 Findings

In this chapter, the main findings of the qualitative research are presented, focusing on how older adults adapt their everyday eating practices to changed life circumstances. Despite various obstacles, resilient participants were determined to maintain independence, continuity and the standard of eating to which they were accustomed and which aligned with social norms. Resilience strategies manifested in all cases, were always shaped by gender and consistently aimed at independence and autonomy. The analysis revealed that resilience is expressed not only in food choice, cooking or food sharing but also in the broader context of social relationships, gender differences and subjectively perceived limitations. Several key themes of dietary resilience emerged: mindful eating and the joy of food, adaptation of eating practices to change, diversification of food sources, use of supportive social networks and knowledge and application of healthy eating principles. The findings are therefore organised around these thematic areas, which gradually reveal how participants cope with the everyday challenges of ageing, health and the social environment.

5.2.1 Autonomy and Independence

Independence was the primary goal towards which all participants[3] aspired. To achieve this goal, they drew on their personal resources related to food and eating.

> I actually quite like it when I feel a bit self-sufficient and independent. (K7MW-SES3)

Some participants with higher socioeconomic status (SES 1–5) said that financial independence allows them to maintain the level of eating they are used to.

> We can still afford to keep our independence and just hope it lasts as long as possible. (K8FSMar-SES1)
> It's not a problem as long as we're mobile and can afford it. Those are the two most important things. (K23MS-SES1)

On the contrary, a lack of individual resources significantly limited both the sense of self-sufficiency and the ability to overcome obstacles.

[3] The participant's code, gender, marital status and SES are provided for each citation.

> I just go to the store, and if there's, like, a discount on something that doesn't look too bad, I'll grab it. But if I feel like having something, I just buy a little bit and get it, you know. Yeah, I wish I had more money so I could buy more veggies. (K1FW-SES7)

Interviews with participants indicated that autonomy is a central goal of their dietary practices, serving as a key motivator when adapting eating behaviours. The ability to independently plan, shop for and prepare meals functioned as an important resilience mechanism, reinforcing a sense of autonomy and control over daily life. Individuals with higher SES had greater capacity to maintain their usual eating standards, whereas limited personal resources constrained their ability to overcome obstacles. This relationship supports resilience theory, which emphasises that adaptive capacity is contingent upon the availability of resources.

5.2.2 Gendered Food Performativity

The interviews revealed that most respondents continue to uphold their gendered roles. Married women considered it highly important to maintain responsibility for all food-related activities as they had traditionally done, ensuring both the continuity of gender roles and the preservation of established standards of dietary practices.

> He likes those old-school foods from his youth, like potato pancakes and stuff. So if I'm feeling nice, I make'em,'cause I'm not that crazy about'em myself. Yeah, I kinda go with what he wants. He's from a conservative family, and I guess I am too, but he's from a super-conservative family. (K5FMar-SES2)

Married men also considered it essential to maintain their habitual dietary practices, typically relying on their partner for meal preparation.

> All the stuff that goes with cooking and eating, like washing the dishes, that's all on the wife. (K19MMar-SES7)

> In the evening, my wife gets everything ready—onions, oil, a bit of salt, adds garlic, stirs it, finishes it off, and by the next day, it's ready. The next day, she puts it all in the roaster when we bake, yeah, and she makes the schnitzel. (K21MMar-SES2)

Due to widowhood or divorce, older adults living alone responded to their circumstances in diverse ways. In most cases, women adapted to the new conditions and developed individual dietary resilience mechanisms to maintain independence. Women living alone did not cook regularly and often prepared meals in advance for future consumption.

> I usually cook enough for, like, three days, which I really like,'cause the next day I don't have to cook. (K6FW-SES4)
> 'Cause I'm mostly at home alone now or just with my boyfriend, I cook what I like, not what maybe other people in the household would like. (K15FW-SES1)

Most men living alone relied on family members or paid help to maintain the dietary intake to which they were accustomed. This difference may be related to lifelong gender role divisions, whereby men are generally not accustomed to independently managing their food practices (Carcedo-Argüelles et al., 2024).

> I get my main meals from my daughter. Every week, she brings me food for the whole week, so I just heat it up. I can manage not to burn it. I have a microwave, so I use that. (K4MW-SES1)
> I don't know how to cook anything… My wife always did everything, and I never even tried to learn. But I can make spaghetti with meat, like Bolognese—that's the only thing. If I happen to be on my own, I can make that for myself. Other than that, I don't cook at all. I don't know how, and I don't even try. (K23MS-SES1)

The findings indicate that older adults often maintain traditional gender roles in food-related practices, with women predominantly responsible for meal preparation and men relying on their partner or external support. Differences between independently living women and men illustrate how gender norms shape opportunities for resilience. The empirical data support the concept of gendered resilience, whereby social roles and culturally conditioned expectations inform adaptive strategies.

In the domain of dietary resilience, five key themes were identified: (i) mindful eating and the enjoyment of food, (ii) adapting dietary practices to changes, (iii) diversification of food sources, (iv) the utilisation of supportive social networks and (v) knowledge and application of healthy eating principles.

5.2.3 Mindful Eating and the Enjoyment of Food

The majority of participants (14) embraced mindful eating and enjoyment of eating as a strategy. They emphasised the importance of enjoying food, savouring it and dedicating more time to meals than they did while working. They decided that good-quality food would be a priority, including financially, and were willing to pay more for high-quality ingredients. The significance of mindful eating and gaining pleasure from eating varied among participants, reflecting the conceptual diversity of dietary resilience. For some, it meant eating according to health-promoting goals, whereas for others it meant consuming foods that provided enjoyment. Both good health and pleasure were identified as primary motivations for their decisions. Resilient individuals were not merely passive recipients of favourable circumstances, they actively took steps to maintain or improve their eating habits in ways that aligned with what enjoying food meant to them (Vesnaver & Keller, 2011). When confronted with specific dietary challenges, they developed resilience strategies to overcome obstacles while preserving mindful eating and its enjoyment. Resilient participants actively sought to sustain this strategy, which also involved creating a pleasant eating environment. Careful meal planning was an integral component, ensuring a variety of protein sources, vegetables and diverse food preparation methods.

> I look forward to breakfast, to be honest, yeah. I still enjoy it. (K4MW-SES1)
> I get pleasure from food. When it's good, it makes me happy. (K20MMar-SES3)

> We definitely enjoy our food. The older we get, the more we enjoy it. (K5FMar-SES2)
> I savour it. I like food, so I enjoy it. I cook what I like, so I enjoy it. For breakfast, for about forty years now, I've had different kinds of bread and various cheeses, and strong dark tea with milk. And I listen to Classic [Praha] radio because it gives me a beautiful, calm morning. (K1FW-SES7)
> I eat at set times. I've always eaten like this. (K11FW-SES1)
> When I plan my food, like when something is cooked or I cook it, I look forward to it like a meal because I know what it will be like. Not that we live just to eat. But tomorrow there'll be dumplings, meat ones. You just count on that… Yeah, some cabbage too. We'll have that. (K10MMar-SES5)
> We cook lunch based on what we feel like. We also switch it up so it's not always potatoes or dumplings or rice or pasta or always meat. Maybe once a week, we'll have something fried. (K18FMar-SES4)

For some participants, the enjoyment experience extended beyond food consumption to related activities such as shopping, with several reporting that they deliberately sought out foods they found pleasurable.

> I go to the store. And I really like buying Csaba sausage. I go to Makro and grab a kilo. (K4MW-SES1)

For them, pleasure was also derived from adhering to the principles of proper dining etiquette, consciously managing both their social and physical eating environments to secure or enhance the enjoyment of food.

> I'm pretty into having a routine, and I like the whole culture and look of food. What I really enjoy is a proper, leisurely breakfast. Honestly, I don't really care if someone's here with me or if I'm on my own. It's just the dining culture. (K7MW-SES3)
> At home, we always ate together, at least when Mom was off work, and we'd look forward to it and talk while eating, so for me it's definitely a ritual. (K17FW-SES1)
> But I always made sure it looked nice. If it's ready, it has to look good on the plate. I can't just dump it there. (K1FW-SES7)

Resilient individuals maintained an active interest in food and its related activities, deliberately seeking out new food items in stores, experimenting with new dishes in restaurants and exploring novel recipes.

> Well, like I said, I mostly follow video recipes, and otherwise, we cook from cookbooks. (K20MMar-SES3)
> I use my partner's son, who's really a foodie, and he knows all the cool places in Prague. When we go together, I'm happy because I get to try something new. (K7MW-SES3)
> It's different in winter and summer. For example, in summer, I don't really crave goulash. When it's hot, it's more like salads or pasta… That's something we both really liked in Italy, whether it was a week in Florence or a week in Venice. We liked things like creamy risotto or pasta with all kinds of little seafood, and, of course, wine, which in Italy is just normal. That's something we grew fond of. (K12MMar-SES5)
> I have files on my computer with recipes. So if I don't know what to cook, I open them and get ideas. I rarely follow the recipe exactly, but I use it as inspiration. (K1FW-SES7)
> When I cook, I like to watch… Classic stuff, like Sapík, because he can cook anything, and it seems really good to me. But those new trends with Thai dishes that need twenty ingredients, I don't even know. I wouldn't know how it's supposed to taste, so I just go out and get them once in a while. (K5FMar-SES2)

Those of our participants who had not developed a resilience mechanism related to mindful eating and enjoyment of food explained this in the following way:

> I eat it just to stay alive. Except for honey. That honey, yeah. (K3FD-SES8)
> I figure food shouldn't be the centre of life, and now it's such a simple thing. So if you just manage it and abide by it, you've got time for other stuff. (K13FW-SES3)
> Of course, sometimes there's food I look forward to, that I really feel like eating, but it definitely doesn't control me. (K7MW-SES3)

Most participants considered enjoyment of food and mindful eating to be key elements of their resilience, both in selecting and preparing meals and in maintaining a high-quality eating environment and dining rituals. Strategies included meal planning, seeking new foods and sustaining enjoyment during eating. These findings support the theoretical framework of resilience, which emphasises active adaptation and the capacity to preserve meaningful daily activities despite limitations.

5.2.4 Adapting to Changes in Dietary Practices

The enjoyment of food thus enabled participants to maintain a positive relationship with eating despite obstacles. Adapting the physical environment to changed health and socioeconomic conditions represented another important resilience mechanism. This primarily involved using various kitchen tools or appliances; purposefully reorganising the kitchen, including furniture rearrangement; or substituting a spoon for cutlery. Participants adjusted both cooking and food consumption to their health status, being acutely aware of the importance of comfort for the eating experience.

> I've got all sorts of stuff in there: a mixer, a kneader, a grater…. (K16MD)
> I just use a spoon or a fork. I can't use a knife now'cause this hand doesn't move, so I just can't. (K2FW-SES8)
> I've got a dishwasher, so I just turn around on the chair, put it in, and once a week or every two weeks, I run it so someone cleans it for me. (K4MW-SES1)

Part of this resilience strategy also involved modifying recipes to make preparation easier. Some participants reported a return to simple meals they remembered from childhood.

> During the week, I usually cook something really simple, most of the time without meat. (K1FW-SES7)
> I make meals that don't take too long'cause I don't feel like spending too much time on them. (K12MMar-SES5)

Some participants simplified meal preparation by cooking two to three days in advance and reheating the food as needed. Preparing larger portions at once to cover multiple meals reduced the daily burden associated with cooking. Participants also froze food, particularly ingredients obtained through self-provisioning.

> I usually don't cook just for one day, I always make enough for at least two, so then I just reheat it. I've got a microwave for that... To be honest, sometimes it's even one of those instant soups from a packet, the three-minute ones. (K3FD-SES1)
> When I'm at home, I cook at home. I normally cook in advance, put everything into containers—soup and the main dish too—and then I just reheat it later. (K15FW-SES1)
> If there's a discount, we'll buy two pork legs, process them, clean them, portion them, freeze them... [In the garden I grow] garlic, onions, tomatoes, peppers, kohlrabi... what else is there? Cucumbers, Hokkaido squash? Beans too. Some of it, we preserve in jars. (K10MMar-SES5)

Participants adapted their shopping strategies to minimise the physical strain of grocery shopping. They often visited multiple stores, making smaller purchases at shorter intervals to avoid carrying heavy bags. Some also used online grocery delivery services or obtained meals from nearby canteens, such as workplaces or schools.

> We go shopping more often, but just for smaller things. We can't carry much anymore. (K5FMar-SES2)
> Most of the stuff I need for the household, if I'm missing something, I just buy it from online shops. (K12MMar-SES5)

Knowledge of culinary techniques and active cooking skills is crucial for enabling older adults to adapt the meals they prepare to age-related changes in taste, digestion and sensory perception.

> Stuffed potato dough and little pockets filled with plum jam, then you drizzle some rum on'em and sprinkle poppy seeds. But that's a Jewish dish that came from Moravia'cause the Jews there grew plums. (K17FW-SES1)

> Apples go on the bottom, sprinkle sugar under'em, and put cinnamon on top. Then, more cinnamon and sugar on the apples. On top of that goes the dough, with two or three eggs, about a cup and a half of flour, half a litre or so, a whole stick of butter, sugar, flour and eggs. Mix it all together and just pour it over. (K16MD)

Resilient participants consumed smaller and/or more frequent meals. Changes in eating habits were observed, such as eating more slowly or taking a walk after meals to facilitate digestion.

> Now I'm finding I can't even eat a whole schnitzel, you know? So most of the time, when I've got it, I just take half of it with me. (K4MW-SES1)
> Smaller portions, depending on what I feel like, that's how I do it. (K12MMar-SES5)

One of the most frequently emphasised changes reported by participants was the regularity of meals.

> And the biggest changes… I'd say regularity for sure. Healthy cooking, none of that half-prepared stuff, no ready meals, none of that—everything I make at home—and also picking good ingredients. Everything's gotten better. (K5FMar-SES2)
> Meals should be regular. That's how it's supposed to be from childhood. (K17FW-SES1)
> Well, I start in the morning around nine… sometimes later, because I stick to twelve hours without eating at night. So the last thing I eat in the evening is before nine, and then breakfast is around nine, and I eat a lot, seriously. (K3FD-SES1)
> I'd say this: I eat when I'm hungry, but I keep a certain regularity 'cause it's good for you. (K13FW-SES3)

Participants employed various strategies to adapt their eating practices to changes in health status and living conditions, including using assistive devices, modifying recipes, planning shopping planning and maintaining regular meal patterns. These strategies demonstrate that resilience manifests not only in the ability to maintain dietary quality but also in flexibility and the capacity to actively adjust daily routines. The findings support the theoretical framework of resilience, which posits that adaptive capacities encompass not only available resources but also practical solutions to constraints and the maintenance of autonomy.

5.2.5 Diversification of Food Sources

Food source diversification represents a significant component of dietary resilience strategies among older adults, as it enhances their capacity to adapt to changes, constraints or crises that may affect food availability, quality or preparation. Older individuals may face barriers such as limited mobility, illness, loss of a driving licence or the closure of nearby stores. Diversifying food sources serves as an adaptive strategy that mitigates the impact of these limitations. When older adults have access to multiple sources, they can move more flexibly between them, combining shopping at brick-and-mortar stores with purchases at markets or online. They may also dine in restaurants or canteens and engage in self-provisioning if they can access a garden.

> We go to a restaurant maybe three, four times a year. (K11FW-SES1)
> There's this chilled-food shop nearby. Pretty handy, so I just go there and usually grab a couple of meals (K11FW-SES1).
> We order online quite often. Down the street in one of the apartment buildings, there's a little shop that sells farm-fresh stuff. We always order through the internet and pay online too. (K12MMar-SES5)
> It's been about two years since we started getting lunch from the public canteen. Here's the menu—don't really pick much, usually just go for the first meal. (K14FMar-SES5)

Due to financial constraints imposed by a fixed but limited pension, our participants actively engaged in self-provisioning, a practice with a strong tradition in the Czech Republic. They cultivated vegetables, fruits and herbs in gardens or on balconies and, frequently, went into forests to collect mushrooms, wild berries and similar resources.

> We've got cherries, and last year, we had tomatoes and cucumbers. So we were thrilled 'cause they were ours and, of course, the best. And strawberries, but that's about it (K5FMar-SES2).
> I've got a garden, loads of currants, so I make currant juice. Pretty much all year, I either drink currant juice or sweeten my tea with it, or make it warm, so in the mornings, I have that hot juice instead of tea. (K6FW-SES4)

Diversifying food sources enables older adults to control their diet despite limited mobility, health issues or financial constraints. Combining shopping in stores, dining at restaurants, ordering online, using public canteens and self-provisioning increases their flexibility and supports autonomy. This mechanism demonstrates that dietary resilience encompasses the capacity to actively utilise available resources and minimise the risk of reduced autonomy.

5.2.6 Mobilising Supportive Social Networks

The boundaries between the food source diversification and the utilisation of supportive social networks are not rigid but rather complementary. Nevertheless, describing these two dietary resilience strategies separately was considered appropriate. In cases where participants were unable to secure their own food, resilient individuals sought assistance from family members and friends and, in some instances, even from neighbours. This support encompassed help with grocery shopping, meal preparation and related tasks, but it also included sharing the meals themselves.

> If we tell [the kids], they're really willing to bring everything over. We don't have the slightest problem with that—they try to help us not just with food, but with other stuff too. I think we're really lucky, the relationships are really good. (K5FMar-SES2)
> Tea, coffee—that's just on weekends. [My daughter] makes cappuccino. Amazing. Otherwise, I can't even lift the kettle to make tea myself. So [my grandson] makes me tea, and then I just drink water. Since my grandson's

> here, he usually makes lunch. And a neighbour comes by, and one day a week we have lunch together. So we usually figure out what we're going to do. (K17FW-SES1)

Commensality is highly significant for older adults, and attitudes toward sharing meals were also included as one of the questions in the questionnaire. Commensality strengthens social cohesion and constitutes an element of resilience both practically and symbolically. This proposition was confirmed by participants' responses, which broadly expressed a desire not to eat alone. It was important for participants to share meals with family or friends, that is, with people to whom they had close relationships. In many cases, meal sharing also occurred in the opposite direction, with women in our sample preparing food for others—not only for their partners but also for other family members, primarily children and grandchildren.

> I usually have lunch with my neighbour every day, and on weekends, with my family. (K17FW-SES1)
> Of course, I prefer eating with someone else or in a group. (K1FW-SES7)
> On Sundays, I always go to my daughter's for lunch. She also invites her daughter, my granddaughter, and her boyfriend, so it's like a big Sunday meal together. (K3FD-SES8)
> The two of us like eating together, and we enjoy inviting friends to eat with us. Or grandchildren. I make the things they like too—pancakes when they're on holiday, for example. (K5FMar-SES2)
> I like eating with company. Yeah, it's important. It's kind of a ritual. (K17FW-SES1)
> I prefer eating with the people closest to me—who else would I eat with? (K10MMar-SES5)
> I cook for my son every other day. (K11FW-SES1)
> At Christmas, [...] Grandpa has to make the soup, beef broth, because the boys only want Grandpa's soup and Grandpa's schnitzels. (K19MMar-SES7)
> We live on a short little street. One neighbour noticed that even though it's small, we don't really know each other. So twice a year, spring and autumn, we have a little get-together. Another neighbour has a nice big yard, partly covered, so that's where we always meet those two times a year. (K12MMar-SES5)

However, several exceptions were also noted in this context.

> I don't really care whether I eat alone or with company. Mostly, I eat with my dad at lunch, and otherwise, I have dinner by myself. (K11FW-SES1)
> I don't mind eating alone. I'm an only child, so I'm used to it, and it doesn't bother me. (K9FS-SES5)

The use of supportive social networks demonstrates that dietary resilience is not solely an individual strategy but also has a pronounced collective dimension. Practical assistance with shopping and cooking is intertwined with commensal practices, which reinforce a sense of belonging and meaningfulness. This strategy thus confirms that resilience is shaped not only by an individual's capacity to adapt but also by the quality of relationships and social support within the community.

5.2.7 Knowledge and Practice of Healthy Eating

The application of healthy eating principles and informed food choices constitutes a key resilience strategy. The majority of resilient participants (18) adhered conscientiously to these principles. Within this framework, participants were willing to pay a premium for high-quality foods or purchase organic products. Food choices were made to prevent potential health issues, adapting them to their individual health conditions. Others emphasised the importance of self-discipline and listening to one's body, particularly in relation to weight management. Participants monitored their weight carefully, especially those with diabetes. Weight management in connection with health status was observed in sixteen participants and was associated with knowledge of their diagnosis and the corresponding dietary requirements.

> I think over the last few years I've been leaning more toward healthy eating. When I was on my own, well, a guy on his own kinda just ignores that stuff. But then, of course, the illness changed my eating when I was in the hospital for heart surgery. And mostly the sugars—that's really dangerous, more dangerous than fats. So, I hold back, 'cause I figure that would make me gain weight. (K12MMar-SES5)

I try to buy healthier stuff now, take more veggies, buy an avocado, maybe some nuts too. And, yeah, don't eat too much sugar. Gotta watch the weight and the sugar. I never had much trouble with my weight, but if I eat sweets, I notice it. (K15FW-SES1)
I think I eat healthy because, for example, I don't buy pork belly, so I figure that's healthy. (K9FS-SES5)
I'd drink wine, but I'd rather have water, or mineral water, unfortunately. Of course, I'd drink wine if I could. (K17FW-SES1)
For the last twenty years, ever since my heart surgery, just diabetes and stuff, I eat breakfast regularly. Before that, I didn't eat breakfast at all. (K19MMar-SES7)
I really have to control myself so I don't gain weight. Even at this age I still have to hold back with food. I eat well in the morning, also at lunch, and in the evening, I'd rather not eat, 'cause that would be bad. (K14FMar-SES3)
You've gotta know your own body, because if you understand it, it'll tell you. I'm not really hungry, so why stuff myself? I watch the fats, try not to have too much. Like, I don't pour fat on my potatoes, I leave them dry, and maybe have some compote, cucumber salad or veggies with it. (K13FW-SES3)
I do try to make the food healthy, so I focus on variety, eat plenty of veggies and try not to make it too fatty because I have high cholesterol. It has to be made from good, healthy ingredients. Can't have anything really harmful in it. (K7MW-SES3)
I don't buy processed foods, or only very rarely. Healthy food for me is food I cook from basic ingredients. I won't cut anything out of my diet—meat, vegetables, all of it. (K8FMar-SES1)
If it's necessary to change the diet for health reasons, well, you just gotta do it. We've reduced portion sizes a bit—they're relatively small now, because that's enough—but otherwise we eat the same stuff. (K12MMar-SES)

Some participants (5) did not adhere to medical advice and preferred to eat without regard for the prescribed diet.

Back in the day, I had an idea of how much I should weigh, and when it started getting worse, I just gave up. And back then, my husband

> was diagnosed with type 2 diabetes, and he started eating super disciplined. He skipped hard liquor, beer, bread... He lost weight 'cause people praised him, and after that, it all went downhill. And I'm not the type to starve myself—I'd get grumpy... I'm not gonna stress. I just wanna enjoy the rest of my life. (K1FW-SES7)
>
> No, seriously, I think the diabetologists were wrong. I eat everything. I eat sweets, chocolate, but I keep moving. I admit, exercise is super important, and I say if you spend at least an hour a day on your body, sugar won't hurt you. (K4MW-SES1)
>
> Well, I've got high cholesterol, shouldn't be eating animal fats. And I do, I'm not disciplined there. (K8F1-SES1)
>
> And I like pork cracklings too. That's probably why my eyes are bad, 'cause I've got sclerosis, but I say, hey, I won't be here forever anyway, so what. I love beer, that's it. I go out with friends for a beer, and we have some wine too. (K6FW-SES4)
>
> As a diabetic, I shouldn't even be eating, I dunno, an apple at five or six o'clock, none of that fruit stuff. But I just say, 'Heck, how long am I gonna be here anyway', and I eat it. (K22MD-SES2)

Interviews with participants demonstrated that older adults employ various dietary strategies that enable them to maintain health, well-being and social embeddedness despite the changes and limitations associated with ageing. These strategies include not only a mindful and enjoyable approach to eating but also flexible adaptation of their diet to current health status and living conditions. Food source diversification plays a significant role, from self-sufficiency and shopping at markets or online to utilising restaurants or meal services. Social support from family, friends and neighbours is also crucial, often encompassing practical assistance, meal sharing and commensal dining. Principles of healthy eating were applied in practice in two ways: for some participants, they involved discipline and control, whereas for others, they entailed adopting a more relaxed approach that allowed them to maintain quality of life and the enjoyment of food. These strategies should not be understood in isolation but rather as interconnected and mutually reinforcing forms of resilience whereby older adults balance tradition, health recommendations and their own needs.

5.3 Discussion

5.3.1 Discussion[4] Overview

From an anthropological perspective, dietary resilience among older adults can be understood as a culturally and biographically anchored mechanism shaped through interaction between historically acquired eating habits, current constraints and societal expectations. This mechanism is not static and evolves alongside life events and structural conditions (Vesnaver et al., 2012).

Prior individual experiences with food form the foundation of each person's dietary patterns and significantly influence current food choices and meal preparation methods among older adults. Their dietary trajectories can persist across life transitions due to the inertia of repeated food choices and ingrained eating habits (Whitelock & Ensaff, 2018). In this context, from an anthropological standpoint, food-related rituals are essential for maintaining cultural continuity and emotional resilience in later life, as they provide both structural stability and psychological support during periods when biological capacities or social ties are weakened (Plastow et al., 2015).

Dietary rituals in later life serve as a means to maintain identity, resilience and cultural continuity. This phenomenon is supported by a systematic review demonstrating that food-related activities directly contribute to the preservation of gender, ethnic and community identities and that changes in these activities, for instance, due to poor health, may threaten individual identity (Plastow et al., 2015). Food-related rituals are not mere routines, they are anchored in memory and carry significant emotional and symbolic meaning. '*I savour it. I like food, so I enjoy it. I cook what I like, so I enjoy it. For breakfast, for about forty years now, I've had different kinds of bread and various cheeses, and strong dark tea with milk. And I listen to Classic* [Praha] *radio because it gives me a beautiful, calm morning' (K1FW-SES7).* This account illustrates how everyday eating routines are not merely practical acts but also serve as

---

[4] Given the focus of the study, it is important to note that the discussion is grounded in the integration of anthropological and nutrition-sociological perspectives.

a means of preserving and re-experiencing personal and cultural history through tastes, smells and sounds. It is in this context that Holtzman (2006) emphasises how food functions as a form of 'embodied memory', linking sensory experiences with memories and life experiences.

For our participants, eating rituals were particularly important in coping with loss, illness or changes in social roles. The transcription and continuation of family recipes, recalling tastes from youth or maintaining the tradition of baking Christmas foods were observed in nearly all interviews. These activities provided respondents not only with a sense of continuity but also with an emotional refuge during life crises (Locher et al., 2005). Gender differences in these rituals are reflected in the ways men and women sustain themselves. Women often bear the responsibility for maintaining traditions through the informal transmission of recipes, baking for the family or organising rituals that reinforce their sense of purpose and social connectedness (Macht et al., 2005). Men, on the other hand, derive a sense of identity from nostalgia for home-cooked flavours, such as their mother's cuisine or family celebratory meals. These nostalgic recollections can serve to express the continuity of their role and meaning. *'Apples go on the bottom, sprinkle sugar under'em, and put cinnamon on top. Then, more cinnamon and sugar on the apples. On top of that goes the dough, with two or three eggs, about a cup and a half of flour, half a litre or so, a whole stick of butter, sugar, flour and eggs. Mix it all together and just pour it over' (K16MD).*

The thematisation of dietary resilience in this study confirms that resilience is shaped by individual determinants, such as the motivation associated with food, and collective determinants, including food availability and social support. This is similarly supported by Payette and Shatenstein (2005), who identified individual factors (health status, personal history) and collective factors (access to food, community support) as the key determinants of healthy eating. Moreover, dietary diversity has been positively associated with psychological resilience in older populations, as shown by Yin et al. (2019). Finally, the qualitative NuAge study (Vesnaver et al., 2012) illustrates how older adults overcome barriers to eating through personal agency and available resources, highlighting the specific interaction between individual and collective resilience mechanisms.

In our empirical research, participants experienced and perceived food and eating in diverse ways. Health and enjoyment were primary considerations for many. Conversely, some participants regarded meals merely as fuel, with their primary purpose to sustain life. The value and meaning of food clearly depended on gender, social relationships, cultural context and the participants' economic situation. Many described how the significance of food and meals had changed compared to earlier life stages, when they were still working and unable to eat regularly or healthily. All participants reported that, in their view, their eating habits improved after retirement. At that point, most began to appreciate mindful eating and to actively seek and derive pleasure from their meals.

For the participants, maintaining independence and control over what they ate was of critical importance. This aligns with findings by Vesnaver et al. (2012), who reported that having control over food and the eating situation was key for the development of dietary resilience. Differences among participants in achieving control over their diets were determined by their levels of autonomy and agency, as well as by the quantity and quality of the resources they could mobilise. These differences, in turn, shaped the areas in which older adults could develop and implement dietary strategies. Jensen et al. (2019) further note that strategies related to food and the eating environment are closely linked not only to individual circumstances but also to participants' personal preferences.

The following sections of the discussion therefore focus in greater detail on the gender framework and specific dietary resilience strategies.

5.3.2 Interpreting Gendered Performativity

In the context of older adults' everyday eating practices, food choices can be understood as performances through which individuals embody and express culturally shared notions of what is proper or appropriate. These performances occur at the level of stated values and are enacted through specific dietary practices. They are deeply gendered and learned, as both men and women acquire lifelong habits of eating in accordance with gendered roles (Lupton, 1996; Plastow et al., 2015). Women are often socialised into caregiver and gendered housekeeper positions through cooking and caring for others, whereas men are guided toward autonomy and an emphasis on pleasure and/or independence, which is reflected in their approaches to food (Counihan, 1999; Brettin et al., 2024).

Our married female respondents confirmed gendered behaviours in the role of caregiver and provider of food, largely guided by their husband's preferences regarding the menu, preparation methods and timing of meals. One participant stated, *'He* [my husband] *likes those old-school foods from his youth, like potato pancakes and stuff. So if I'm feeling nice, I make'em, 'cause I'm not that crazy about'em myself. Yeah, I kinda go with what he wants. He's from a conservative family, and I guess I am too, but he's from a super-conservative family' (K5FMar-SES2).* Such continuations of established gender roles can be understood as a resilience mechanism, as they represent a way for married women to affirm their caregiver role and maintain its continuity.

Most single women in our sample adapted their lives to new circumstances and developed individual dietary resilience mechanisms to maintain independence. One participant stated: *'Because I'm mostly at home alone now or just with my boyfriend, I cook what I like, not what maybe other people in the household would like' (K15FW-SES1).* This woman, after widowhood, clearly welcomed the opportunity to adapt her diet to her own needs.

Generally, older women tend to adhere more closely to medical dietary recommendations. Evidence from the literature indicates that older women are more likely to comply with prescribed diets (Kearney et al., 2002). In contrast, older men often respond to medical oversight with resistance, perceiving it as infantilising or as a threat to their masculine identity and independence, and are reluctant to follow recommendations they consider unnecessary or restrictive (Rose et al., 2024). Some respondents did not adopt the recommended dietary changes due to stereotypical notions of personal freedom, enjoyment of food or control: 'A*s a diabetic, I shouldn't even be eating, I dunno, an apple at five or six o'clock, none of that fruit stuff. But I just say, "Heck, how long am I gonna be here anyway," and I eat it' (K22MD-SES2).* Such behaviour can be understood as a performance of independence and resistance to medical authority, expressed through masculine notions of autonomy (Mahalik et al., 2007). Both men and women negotiate between personal taste, cultural habits and medical authority. This is further supported by systematic reviews of Mediterranean diet intervention studies, which show that women demonstrate slightly higher adherence. In contrast, men's motivation to follow dietary recommendations is shaped by their perceptions of their role and their bodies (Rose et al., 2024).

The experience of ageing, food and care should thus be understood as a space for identity reflection, where individuals not only satisfy their needs but also communicate values, relationships and cultural embeddedness, often through gender-structured food practices. Choices and activities related to food can express group membership, reinforce cultural values and evoke memories that shape self-concept. Conversely, changes in eating habits due to health conditions or other life events may disrupt this sense of identity (Plastow et al., 2015).

Older adults must navigate changing dietary needs and physical limitations while gendered beliefs regarding food, body image and health persist. Women may face pressure to consume 'light' meals and maintain a slender physique, whereas men may resist dietary restrictions that conflict with notions of masculinity and autonomy. Weight management was a concern for all our participants, particularly those with diabetes. Among women, attention to weight was closely linked to knowledge of their diagnosis and adherence to prescribed dietary regimens: '*I really have to control myself so I don't gain weight. Even at this age, I still have to hold back with food. I eat well in the morning, also at lunch, and in the evening, I'd rather not eat, 'cause that would be bad' (K14FMar-SES3).*

Ageing in later life is not merely a biological process but a deeply culturally mediated experience that profoundly shapes everyday food practices. The body cannot be understood solely as an object of physiological decline but as a cultural space through which norms, values and identities are expressed and experienced (Scheper-Hughes & Lock, 1987). Changes in physical capacities, such as the loss of taste, smell or mobility, are not perceived merely as bodily impairments but carry moral and symbolic meanings that are shaped throughout life in accordance with gendered roles (Lupton, 1996). Women, who often bear lifelong responsibility for feeding others, tend to be particularly attentive to adjusting their diets for health purposes: '*I don't buy processed foods, or only very rarely. Healthy food for me is food I cook from basic ingredients.*

I won't cut anything out of my diet—meat, vegetables, all of it' (K8FMar-SES1). Men, on the other hand, may perceive bodily decline as a threat to their traditionally masculine identity (Plastow et al., 2015) Food in later life does not merely serve as a means of nutrition but becomes a tool through which individuals interpret bodily changes, renegotiate their identity and maintain or challenge prior roles and expectations (Oleschuk, 2019). This process is always embedded within a broader cultural context that defines what constitutes 'good food', 'proper ageing' and a 'cared for body'. In relation to body image, older women are often defined as sexually unattractive and inactive, judged against ideals of female beauty that emphasise youthfulness and thinness. This ideal renders ageing a potentially humiliating process of sexual disqualification (Marshall, 2017). In contrast, older men's experiences are less closely tied to physical attractiveness; they may be valued for associations between maturity and socially prized 'masculine' attributes, such as power or wealth (Twig, 2013).

The reduction in food consumption observed among our participants carries significant gendered connotations. Older women may interpret a decreased appetite as a natural aspect of ageing and associate it with ideals of femininity, restraint and moral self-control internalised over the life course (Lupton, 1996). Conversely, older men may perceive a loss of appetite or dietary restrictions as a threat to their masculinity—particularly when required to follow diets limiting red meat or alcohol, foods often linked to hegemonic masculinity (Gough & Conner, 2006). Simultaneously, women may continue to avoid 'heavy' foods in later life to conform to culturally entrenched notions of female thinness and lightness (Oleschuk, 2019): *'We eat pretty little, I'd say. I try to watch my weight, but we're not really that hungry anymore, don't feel the need. And I mostly keep an eye on my weight for how I look' (K5FMar-SES2).* Food taboos, restrictions and rituals are thus not neutral, they reflect socially and gender-conditioned notions of what it means to 'age properly', whether as a disciplined and caring woman or as a self-sufficient and strong man (Twigg, 2004).

Our female participants who maintained gardens engaged in gardening practices and processed and preserved their harvests. This finding aligns with anthropological research showing that older women often possess a rich repertoire of intergenerationally transmitted knowledge related to food preparation, seasonal ingredient processing and the use of medicinal herbs. Such knowledge, frequently acquired through everyday household and family care, contributes not only to the food security and health of the women themselves but also to that of their close relatives (Sachs & Patel-Campillo, 2014). These activities are increasingly recognised as forms of cultural and ecological resilience, offering alternatives to industrial food systems and dependence on biomedical care.

In contrast, men may maintain other types of embodied food knowledge, such as hunting, fishing or foraging practices. These activities are often associated with ideals of self-sufficiency, independence and traditional masculine identity, and they too can represent sources of autonomy and meaning in later life (Bye, 2003). Research confirms that both female and male knowledge and skills in subsistence activities, such as gardening, crop gathering or fishing, are not merely relics of the past but significantly contribute to food resilience and the ability to adapt to changing life conditions, health limitations or economic uncertainty. For instance, a systematic review of gendered traditional agroecological knowledge indicates that both sexes possess specialised knowledge: women more often in food preservation and domestic processing, and men primarily in production or field collection activities. This embodied, culturally grounded knowledge is essential for daily food provisioning and survival amid diverse socioeconomic pressures and environmental changes (Ramirez-Santos et al., 2023). One participant remarked, '*I've got a garden, loads of currants, so I make currant juice. Pretty much all year, I either drink currant juice or sweeten my tea with it, or make it warm, so in the mornings, I have that hot juice instead of tea*' *(K6FW-SES4)*. This finding confirms that food resilience is not achievable solely through institutional or market-based support, but also through shared and transmitted knowledge that carries cultural, practical and symbolic significance.

Another way in which older women in our sample—both married and living alone—expressed their resilience was through cooking for others, primarily for family members. In our study, married women considered it natural to care for their husbands and families, and they took pride in the domestic work they performed. In some cases, they consciously reduced their own food intake to ensure that others had enough. However, these practices were not merely economic decisions; they represented a moral performance of femininity and care (DeVault, 1991). Grandparenting served as a means of expressing love through food. Intergenerational relationships, particularly those associated with the roles of grandmother or grandfather, constitute a key domain of gendered performativity in food practices. Among women, this was often manifested as ongoing, regular care and cooking for children and grandchildren: *'I cook for my son every other day' (K11FW-SES1).* Among men, it was evident that they perceived the role of grandfather in relation to food as exceptional and limited to specific occasions: *'Usually white sausage at Christmas or a schnitzel. And Grandpa has to make the soup, beef broth, because the boys only want Grandpa's soup and Grandpa's schnitzels' (K19MMar-SES7).*

Shared meals in later life represent not only a source of nutrition but also a crucial social and symbolic framework through which individuals experience a sense of belonging, identity and daily structure. From an anthropological perspective, eating is a deeply embedded cultural practice, and its disruption can significantly affect wellbeing and resilience (DeVault, 1991; Rueda & Artazcoz, 2009). Research repeatedly shows that older women in particular are more likely to maintain social forms of eating—cooking for others, sharing meals with friends or participating in community meals—which contributes to their psychological and emotional resilience (DeVault, 1991; Vesnaver et al., 2012). One respondent shared the following insight: *'When [my son] comes over, I ask what they want, cause they just expect something different from Grandma than from their mom. "So, Grandma, schnitzels?" Last time they were here, I made a big pot of potato salad and really baked schnitzels for them—one chicken, one pork, fried cauliflower, yeah—and so everyone could take what they liked' (K8FMar-SES1).*

Another perspective frames cooking for others as a form of gift-giving. Among older women, the ethics of care can be expressed through responding to the needs of others, and cooking may be understood as an enactment of a gift (Mol, 2021). The act of giving food is thus closely tied to the feminine role, and the labour associated with cooking can be perceived as producing value within the household. Food consumption as a gift becomes, in this view, the intended outcome of cooking (Sidenvall et al., 2000). Thus, it is understandable that for our widowed respondents, the loss of commensality was experienced as particularly painful, as empirical evidence shows that older women often derive joy from preparing food for others (Abbots & Lavis, 2016). *'The two of us like eating together, and we enjoy inviting friends to eat with us. Or grandchildren. I make the things they like too—pancakes when they're on holiday, for example' (K5FMar-SES2).* Whether it involves gardening, caring for grandchildren or sharing meals as a gift, these practices represent forms of care performativity through which older adults cultivate their dietary resilience. They are united not only by an orientation toward others but also by the capacity to transform everyday activities into a means of reinforcing relationships, identity and meaningfulness.

In contrast, men who age in solitude often face both practical and psychological barriers related to food acquisition, preparation and consumption. Studies indicate that solitary men tend to exhibit lower diet quality, reduced caloric intake and a higher risk of malnutrition. Eating alone is experienced not merely as a practical necessity but also as a loss of the social role previously mediated by a partner or family framework (Locher et al., 2005; Hanna et al., 2023). The absence of shared meals can therefore represent a deeper symbolic uprooting for men, whereas women tend to adapt more flexibly, for instance, through informal meal sharing with friends or neighbours (Vesnaver et al., 2016). In our sample, solitary men, with two exceptions, attempted to compensate for this loss of social role by seeking out relatives—typically daughters—who would prepare and serve meals for them. Those without relatives relied on paid services. This pattern may be linked to lifelong gender role divisions, where men are less accustomed to independently managing their dietary needs (Carcedo-Argüelles et al., 2024). *'I don't know how to cook anything… My wife always did everything, and I never even tried to learn. But I can make spaghetti with meat, like bolognese—that's the only thing. If I happen to be on my own, I can make that for myself. Other than that, I don't cook at all. I don't know how, and I don't even try' (K23MS-SES1).*

Indirectly, we found from married male respondents that, in at least two cases, both partners prepared all their own meals, or at least breakfast and lunch. The remaining married men in our sample continued their previous eating patterns, relying on their wives to maintain established gendered dietary routines, which in later life, often become subjects of negotiation, resistance or reinforcement. Recent studies indicate that women are more likely than men to perceive responsibility for preparing proper meals as a moral obligation, even when facing health or material constraints themselves (Oleschuk, 2019). Conversely, older men frequently contend with a lack of practical cooking skills alongside masculine norms that may complicate adherence to dietary restrictions (Sellaeg & Chapman, 2008). One participant noted, '*I get my main meals from my daughter. Every week, she brings me food for the whole week, so I just heat it up. I can manage not to burn it. I have a microwave, so I use that' (K4MW-SES1).*

The gendered impact of isolation among older men is further corroborated by extensive research from the Japan Gerontological Evaluation Study cohort, which demonstrated that men who eat alone and lack social support face a significantly higher risk of depression and mortality (Tani et al., 2020). Although eating alone is also associated with depressive symptoms among women, it more frequently occurs within a broader spectrum of caregiving activities, such as caring for grandchildren or maintaining neighbourhood networks. '*I usually have lunch with my neighbour every day, and on weekends, with my family' (K17FW-SES1).* Nonetheless, Whitelock and Ensaff (2018) note that a lack of motivation to cook has been observed among older women who have lost a partner, which is significant given that motivation constitutes an influential factor in healthy eating, particularly when cooking for oneself and eating alone.

Gendered performativity in the eating practices of older adults thus oscillates between continuity and change. On the one hand, older women and men build upon lifelong acquired roles: women often through caregiving for others and men through maintaining notions of autonomy and masculinity. On the other hand, in the context of ageing, these roles transform and create space for new forms of resilience. Women may, for instance, seek independence by cooking for themselves, while men may sometimes learn to accept support or acquire new skills.

Gendered performativity in this context can function both as a source of vulnerability—such as in cases of loneliness or the inability to fulfil traditional roles—and as a resource that enhances the meaningfulness of everyday life and fortifies resilience against the challenges of ageing.

5.3.3 The Role of Mindful Eating and Pleasure in Dietary Resilience

Mindful eating is one of the most frequently mentioned resilience strategies in the diets of older adults (Winkens et al., 2018). It involves the deliberate enjoyment of food, associated not only with pleasure derived from the food itself but also from the activities surrounding it. Mindful activities related to eating are performed with the aim of creating meaningful situations (Jensen et al., 2019). Paolini et al. (2012) found that individuals with higher levels of mindfulness exhibited better recovery of functional brain networks, indicating an enhanced ability to regulate responses to food, which may be particularly important for eating behaviours in later life. The literature consistently recognises mindful eating as an effective approach not only against obesity but also against malnutrition in older age (Carrière et al., 2022; Sivri & Yur, 2024). A mindful approach discourages strict dieting and moralising about food choices, promotes attentiveness to bodily cues and, when applied consistently, can improve one's relationship with both food and the body.

In later life, mindful eating and the enjoyment of food are also perceived as sources of independence, identity and overall wellbeing (Plastow et al., 2015): *'I actually quite like it when I feel a bit self-sufficient and independent' (K7MW-SES3).* This connection arises both through sensory engagement with food as well as through the cultural meanings and personal memories associated with specific dishes (Bédard et al., 2020). Among older adults, the relationship between pleasure, memory and place is particularly strong. Flavours from childhood or the aromas of a home kitchen are often linked to feelings of safety, recognition and continuity (Nyberg et al., 2018). According to Moscato and Ozanne (2019), pleasure can also be understood as an act of resistance against dominant discourses of active and 'proper' ageing. At the same time, pleasure is not necessarily at odds with health promotion; on the contrary, it can contribute to it (Plastow et al., 2015).

In our study, the pursuit of pleasure was often anchored not only in the food itself but also in related activities. Of our twenty-three participants, twenty reported enjoyment from eating and/or associated practices. For our participants, pleasure was provided by adherence to principles of good dining: *'I stick to basic table manners, you know, the usual stuff. Plates, two forks and knives, napkins… I set the table properly' (K8FMar-SES1).* The emphasis on table manners illustrates how mindful eating encompasses more than just the act of consumption but also the broader socio-symbolic context of food (Bédard et al., 2020). Pleasure was also derived from grocery shopping: *'I say, yeah, it's more expensive. So, you know, if you've tried it, you get it. But I don't mind at all, because that's exactly it—when I just have bread with butter, for me it's like a treat. No, it's not really worth it money-wise. But, feeling-wise and with the taste and everything, I just prefer to go and buy that pricier bread' (K23MS-SES1).* They also derived pleasure from preparing meals using new recipes or from consuming dishes from foreign cuisines. *'I think, like, traditionally even around the world, Italian food is good or French restaurants. But Asian food is good too' (K15FW-SES1).* An integral component of mindful eating also involved careful meal planning: *'When I plan my food, like when something is cooked or I cook it, I look forward to it like a meal because I know what it will be like. Not that we live just to eat. But tomorrow there'll be dumplings, meat ones. You just count on that… Yeah, some cabbage too. We'll have that' (K10MMar-SES5).*

In older adult populations, validated tools such as the Anticipatory and Consumatory Eating Pleasure Scale have demonstrated that pleasure derived both from anticipating and consuming food is strongly associated with improved appetite, better nutritional status and reduced depressive symptoms (Bailly et al., 2020). Qualitative and model-based studies among older adults in communal dining settings further indicate that positive eating experiences significantly enhance overall wellbeing, particularly when coupled with a sense of group belonging and a pleasant dining environment (Wang et al., 2024).

For the implementation of mindful eating and enjoyment of food as a resilience strategy, culinary knowledge and active cooking skills are essential. These competencies enable older adults to adapt the meals they prepare to changes in taste, digestion and sensory perception associated with ageing: *'Apples go on the bottom, sprinkle sugar under'em, and put cinnamon on top. Then, more cinnamon and sugar on the apples. On top of that goes the dough, with two or three eggs, about a cup and a half of flour, half a litre or so, a whole stick of butter, sugar, flour and eggs. Mix it all together and just pour it over' (K16MD).*

Tani et al. (2020), in a study of the Japanese population aged 65 and older, report that a lack of cooking knowledge is associated with a lower frequency of home-cooked meals, reduced consumption of fruits and vegetables and a higher likelihood of malnutrition, particularly among men. Mastery of culinary skills has significant positive outcomes, including a healthier diet and greater self-sufficiency in food preparation (Reicks et al., 2014). Participants in our study shared descriptions and recipes of their favourite dishes, which allowed us to observe that, with few exceptions, they are culinarily proficient, learn new recipes that better suit their health needs and have a clear understanding of what is best for their wellbeing. The experiences of our participants indicate that mindful eating and culinary competence are not merely survival strategies but active means through which older adults maintain control, purpose and enjoyment in their daily eating practices. Mindful eating integrates sensory pleasure with cultural significance and health benefits, thereby functioning as a strategy that extends beyond mere nutrition, providing older adults with better dietary habits and a sense of continuity, safety and order despite physical or social limitations. In this regard, mindful eating operates as a resilience mechanism, enabling older adults to transform ordinary food-related activities into tools for preserving identity and independence.

5.3.4 Understanding Adaptation to Health and Life Course Changes

The majority of participants in our study adapted their food practices to their health status, being acutely aware of the importance of well-being in eating for their overall health. In doing so, they frequently relied on various kitchen tools and appliances. These aid choices were primarily motivated by the need to compensate for weakened motor abilities, diminished grip strength, reduced physical power or limited reach. *'I just use a spoon or a fork. I can't use a knife now'cause this hand doesn't move, so I just can't' (K2FW-SES8).* Among the most frequently mentioned were ergonomically shaped handles, non-slip mats, electric can and jar openers, food processors facilitating chopping and blending and microwave ovens for convenient meal reheating: *'I usually don't cook just for one day, I always make enough for at least two, so then I just reheat it. I've got a microwave for that' (K3FD-SES1).* The microwave oven, along with other appliances and tools, can, in this context, be regarded as an instrument that supports self-sufficiency rather than merely offering convenience for older adults. Technological adaptation contributes to greater independence in food preparation while simultaneously reducing risk of injury, frustration or resignation from home cooking. As Xu et al. (2024) note, appropriate devices can significantly impact the ability of older adults to maintain nutritional self-sufficiency and, consequently, on overall wellbeing. Similarly, Gagnon-Roy et al. (2022) emphasise that the use of adapted kitchen tools constitutes one of the key factors in promoting food security among individuals with chronic illnesses and functional limitations.

Part of adapting to new circumstances also involves modifying recipes to make them easier to prepare. This represents a common resilience mechanism, as highlighted by Whitelock and Ensaff (2018), who observed that limited physical functioning and manual dexterity often led participants to rely on simple and convenient meals: *'During the week, I usually cook something really simple, most of the time without meat' (K1FW-SES7).*

A common form of adaptation to new circumstances, observed among nearly all participants, was batch cooking several days in advance and reheating meals gradually. This practice reduced the daily burden associated with meal preparation. Participants often froze prepared dishes, particularly foods obtained through self-provisioning. Such a strategy lowered physical strain, minimised the time required for cooking and reduced the cognitive load: *'When I'm at home, I cook at home. I normally cook in advance, put everything into containers—soup and the main dish too—and then I just reheat it later' (K15FW-SES1).* According to Klein and Parks (2020), this mode of eating is particularly advantageous for older adults with limited mobility and chronic illness. The importance of convenient meal preparation, as demonstrated in their study, emerged as a key factor in food choices among older adults who are largely homebound. Many of our participants also reported reduced appetite and lower food intake in later life as reasons for preparing simpler meals. One resulting change in their dietary practices was therefore the consumption of smaller portions. Whitelock and Ensaff (2018), in their qualitative study, likewise note that portion sizes are often too large for older adults and that appetite tends to decline with age. The resilient participants in our research not only consumed smaller portions but also ate more frequently and regularly, with dinner typically taken in the late afternoon rather than in the evening: *'Smaller portions, depending on what I feel like, that's how I do it' (K12MMar-SES5).*

Nyberg et al. (2018) note that participants in their study who experienced motor impairments while eating managed their dietary practices through continuous adjustment and adaptation to the challenges arising from these difficulties. This manifested in the deliberate planning of what and when to eat, the avoidance of certain foods and beverages and the use of simple eating aids.

An interesting finding of our research was that some participants made a conscious decision to eat alone. The primary reason was discomfort or embarrassment associated with wearing dentures: *'I don't mind eating alone. I'm an only child, so I'm used to it, and it doesn't bother me' (K9FS-SES5).* This example demonstrates that resilience in eating need not only rely on actively seeking social interactions, as is often emphasised in the literature (Plastow et al., 2015; Wang et al., 2024), but can also manifest as a strategy of avoidance. As Nyberg et al. (2018) highlight, older adults with motor or health limitations sometimes choose solitary eating in order to maintain control over the situation and to avoid feelings of stigmatisation. This phenomenon can also be interpreted through Goffman's theory of impression management, as eating in social contexts is a socially exposed activity and difficulties in consumption may threaten one's perceived dignity and social 'front' (Goffman, 1959).

From a resilience perspective, eating alone can paradoxically represent an adaptive mechanism that protects an individual's identity and self-esteem (Wiles et al., 2012). This also illustrates a certain ambivalence: whereas communal eating is often understood as a source of wellbeing and a means of preventing social isolation (Wang et al., 2024), for some older adults, it can become a source of stress and perceived threat. Our study's findings thus extend existing knowledge by showing that resilience is not just universally linked to active social participation, but can also manifest as 'defensive' strategies that allow older adults to maintain a sense of autonomy and dignity, even at the cost of reduced social engagement.

All activities aimed at modifying the environment, including tools for food preparation and consumption, were crucial in enabling participants to continue 'appropriate' eating behaviours, maintain a social façade and act in accordance with perceived norms. Food and communal dining were perceived as sources of pleasure as well as a means of maintaining health and a form of 'fuel', whose primary purpose is to sustain life within normal parameters. Our participants similarly managed their dietary practices in this way: '*The biggest changes… I'd say regularity for sure. Healthy cooking, none of that half-prepared stuff, no ready meals, none of that—everything I make at home—and also picking good ingredients. Everything's gotten better' (K5FMar-SES2).*

The findings regarding grocery shopping were also notable. Most participants reported shopping more frequently to avoid carrying heavy bags, while some made use of grocery delivery services. Frequent shopping, however, also carried social significance. The fact that participants went shopping daily and described it as the flexibility to shop whenever they wished is an interesting observation, reflecting the evolving role of grocery shopping in later life. Shopping increasingly acquires a social dimension, maintaining interpersonal interactions—an important factor given the heightened risk of social isolation among older adults (Whitelock & Ensaff, 2018). The changing needs of older adults in relation to age and health status, as well as their impact on dietary practices, are important and warrant further investigation.

Adapting eating practices to shifting health and social conditions thus constitutes a complex set of everyday resilience strategies, enabling older adults to maintain autonomy, reinforce their identity and preserve the continuity of meaningful and dignified eating even in advanced age.

5.3.5 Diversifying Food Sources[5] as a Resilience Strategy

Older adults frequently face a range of barriers, including reduced mobility, chronic illnesses, the loss of their ability to drive, social isolation or the closure of local shops (Tucher et al., 2021; Sharkey, 2008). In this context, food source diversification represents a key resilience strategy. It enables a flexible response to changes, limitations or crises that may negatively impact food availability, quality or preparation. Diversifying food sources is not merely a matter of individual choice but is deeply embedded in structural conditions such as age, health, marital status, gender and socioeconomic status. Older adults' use of multiple food access options reflects not only their adaptive capacity but also cultural norms, social support and access to resources. Our research indicated that physical condition and transportation availability (e.g., car ownership) significantly influence decisions regarding which types of food sources are utilised. Thus, diversification of food sources cannot always be regarded as a matter of free choice; it is often a necessity arising from functional abilities and available resources (Sharkey, 2008).

[5] The boundary between diversifying food sources and utilising support networks is not rigid; rather, these strategies tend to complement one another. Nevertheless, it was considered appropriate to describe these two dietary resilience strategies separately.

The ability to procure food from multiple sources, such as combining in-store shopping with online purchases, emerges as an adaptive strategy that supports self-sufficiency and a sense of control over one's diet (Dean et al., 2009). Participants in our study similarly selected food sources based on their physical capacity and purchasing opportunities: *'Most of the stuff I need for the household, if I'm missing something, I just buy it from online shops' (K12MMar-SES5).* In addition to online shopping, daily or weekly visits to physical stores played an important role. A large proportion of married participants shopped at smaller stores daily, while they undertook larger weekly shopping trips by car. This pattern is also reflected in studies showing that loneliness and social isolation increase vulnerability to food insecurity, whereas cohabitation supports regular eating habits (Locher et al., 2009; Dean et al., 2009). Half of the participants used online grocery shopping, but only two did so on a regular basis. The low frequency of online shopping may reflect generational limitations in digital literacy as well as the concept of foodscapes, which understands the food environment as an economic or logistical framework, but also as a socio-spatial experience (Mikkelsen, 2011). These everyday shopping practices therefore serve to ensure food supply and support social contact, routine and a sense of continuity. From a resilience perspective, this practice can be understood as a strategy that extends beyond physical access to food and strengthens the psychosocial dimension of resilience in older age.

Some older adults also utilise restaurant or community dining, which simultaneously addresses their social needs (Locher et al., 2009). They may also use meal delivery services organised by local municipalities or charitable organisations. In our study, only one married participant used charity-provided food delivery. Married couples visited restaurants infrequently, typically only a few times per year, whereas women living alone with higher socioeconomic status frequented restaurants or cafés regularly, likely not solely for the food but also as a form of social engagement: *'I love beer, that's it. I go out with friends for a beer, and we have some wine too'. (K6FW-SES4).* Among the men living alone, only one reported regularly dining in restaurants. This difference aligns with findings from previous studies showing that men who live independently are particularly vulnerable in terms of nutrition following the loss of a partner, often experiencing poorer dietary intake and making less use of communal eating opportunities (Wills et al., 2011). Thus, the diversification of food sources is not merely an individual adaptation but also reflects culturally embedded gender roles.

Due to financial constraints—stemming from a fixed but limited pension—our participants actively engaged in self-provisioning. This practice constitutes a significant aspect of life for older Czech adults as it both offsets part of their food-related expenses and also supports autonomy, self-confidence, enjoyment and physical activity. Self-provisioning is not unusual in the Czech context as most urban residents have access to a garden, whether through municipal allotment gardens or rural properties, such as cottages or chalets with adjoining land. This phenomenon can be understood as a legacy of historically rooted relationships to land and self-sufficiency, which were further reinforced during the socialist period when self-provisioning was officially encouraged (Gibas et al., 2013). Access to land and knowledge of basic cultivation and processing techniques remain strongly present in the cultural memory of Czech society (Pixová & Plank, 2025).

Beyond the financial dimension, self-provisioning serves a psychosocial function for older adults. Active involvement in growing and processing food can be interpreted as part of an active ageing process, helping seniors avoid passivity while maintaining both physical and mental engagement. This activity fosters a sense of purpose, competence and continuity—values essential for sustaining quality of life in later years (Walker & Maltby, 2012).

The practice of foraging for mushrooms and wild fruits is also deeply rooted in Czech culture, representing both an ecological means of obtaining food and a cultural practice that involves knowledge of nature, seasonality and intergenerational skill transmission (Jehlička et al., 2013). For seniors, gardening and forest foraging function fully as resilience strategies, supporting dignity in later life. Self-provisioning among older adults can also be seen as a form of environmental resilience whereby older individuals utilise local resources and traditional knowledge, enhancing not only food security but also connections with the landscape and community (Veen et al., 2015).

In this context, food source diversification can be understood not only as a means of securing physical access to food but also as a strategy that enhances overall resilience and quality of life in later life (Bowling & Dieppe, 2005). Moreover, it represents a culturally and historically rooted practice that enables older adults to maintain self-sufficiency, fulfil social needs and preserve continuity of identity and values associated with food. From the perspective of resilience theory, diversification can be conceptualised as a form of redundancy, whereby multiple sources perform similar functions so that the failure or loss of one resource strengthens the overall stability of the system (Folke, 2006).

5.3.6 Mobilising Social Networks for Dietary Resilience

Food is a social activity that embodies culture, history and lifestyle (Fischler, 1988). Eating practices are socially conditioned, as they are learned in accordance with shared cultural values and norms, making food preferences and behaviours integral to an individual's social and personal identity (Vesnaver & Keller, 2011). Cultural norms can dictate what is eaten, but also when, how much and with whom. Adherence to established eating practices can further provide a sense of belonging to a particular group. Beyond social roles and culture, social relationships can influence food intake among older adults, who may rely on their social networks for food-related activities such as grocery shopping and meal preparation (Keller, 2006). The social context of food consumption is therefore a crucial consideration in any nutritional research.

In later life, when the need for informal or formal care arises, food becomes a central element through which care is provided. Assistance may initially involve securing groceries and delivering larger shopping orders, progress to sharing or delivering prepared meals and, eventually, extend to full food provision for a family member who can no longer cook independently. In cases where participants in our study were unable to manage their own nutrition, they sought help from family members, friends and, in some instances, neighbours. This assistance primarily included support with grocery shopping, meal preparation and related tasks, as well as shared meal consumption: '*I usually have lunch with my neighbour every day, and on weekends, with my family*'. *(K17FW-SES1)*.

Commensality is highly significant for older adults, and attitudes toward sharing meals were among the questions posed to our participants. The opportunity to share food or cook together is frequently described as an activity that provides meaning and enjoyment (Nyberg et al., 2018). Our participants clearly expressed a preference not to eat alone. It was important for them to share meals with family or friends, that is, with individuals with whom they maintained a close relationship: '*I like eating with company. Yeah, it's important. It's kind of a ritual*' *(K17FW-SES1)*. The social role of food practices within partnered relationships is largely evident from the interviews, as most participants almost invariably discuss food in regard to their partner or, alternatively, other individuals: '*The two of us like eating together, and we enjoy inviting friends to eat with us. Or grandchildren. I make the things they like too*' *(K5FMar-SES2)*. These statements serve to describe how the relationship is perceived and depict mutual similarities, contrasts, disagreements and the interpersonal dynamics of affection, willingness to help, adaptation, evaluation, guidance and so forth (DeVault, 1991).

The diversity of these needs and forms of relationality through food is considerable. The motif of relational dynamics is also reflected in our dataset, where for some respondents the central theme is how they themselves contribute to the younger generation through food—whether by cooking for family members, providing preserved goods or sharing produce from the garden: '*I cook for my son every other day*' *(K11FW-SES1)*. For others, the predominant theme is the reception of assistance from others: '*If we tell* [the kids], *they're really willing to bring everything over. We don't have the slightest problem with that—they try to help us not just with food, but with other stuff too. I think we're really lucky, the relationships are really good*' *(K5FMar-SES2)*.

The interviews suggest that the context of older age amplifies the significance of relationality in eating due to two interrelated circumstances. First, meals are more frequently prepared and consumed at home, thereby providing a structure for the involvement of a partner or other family members (Middleton et al., 2022). Second, eating in later life often serves as a medium for intergenerational relationships of mutual care and support as well as for the maintenance of family ties (Wang et al., 2024). Moreover, social networks are crucial for older adults, as social isolation is recognised as a key predictor of malnutrition risk (Locher et al., 2005; Dean et al., 2009).

Social networking through food thus represents a critical source of resilience for older adults as it provides material support, sustains meaningful relationships and a sense of belonging. Our findings indicate that shared meals, commensality and intergenerational exchanges of care through food foster a sense of belonging and act as a significant resilience mechanism. In line with resilience theory, the use of social networks can be understood as a form of social capital that helps older adults overcome functional limitations, prevent social isolation and maintain quality of life in later life (Bourdieu, 1984).

5.3.7 Applying Nutritional Knowledge in Everyday Food Practices

Resilience strategies in later life often include the selection of healthy foods, which serves as a means to extend both longevity and quality of life, as well as to maintain overall health (Nyberg et al., 2018).

The participants in our study largely adhered strictly to principles of healthy eating, primarily to preserve their health and prevent its deterioration. Food choices were made with consideration of existing health limitations and conditions, functioning as a preventive measure against potential health issues, and diets were planned in accordance with medical recommendations. When procuring healthy foods, participants were willing to incur additional costs and were acutely aware of the potential harms of industrially processed foods. They also sought to allocate sufficient time for meals and to maintain regular eating patterns. *'For the last twenty years, ever since my heart surgery, just diabetes and stuff, I eat breakfast regularly. Before that, I didn't eat breakfast at all' (K19MMar-SES7).* The majority of participants adhered diligently to these dietary rules. This group was well-informed about their health status and appropriate food choices. Our findings confirm that information and education play a crucial role in the dietary practices of older adults. Nutritional literacy is essential for maintaining autonomy and preventing disease in older adults, encompassing knowledge, skills and the ability to apply principles of healthy eating in daily life. Mahony et al. (2023) highlight the need for high-quality nutritional education while Choi et al. (2021), in an American study, demonstrate that improving nutritional literacy through education and marketing is an effective way of enhancing diet quality, food access and social support among older adults. Similarly, Oliveira et al. (2021) underscore the necessity for greater nutritional awareness among older adults, with 69% of seniors in their study expressing a desire for more information about appropriate nutrition.

Half of our study participants monitored their weight, particularly those diagnosed with diabetes. Weight monitoring was associated with awareness of their diagnosis and adherence to a corresponding healthy diet. Participants who followed dietary recommendations were willing to pay extra for high-quality foods or purchased products of organic quality: *'I do try to make the food healthy, so I focus on variety, eat plenty of veggies and try not to make it too fatty because I have high cholesterol. It has to be made from good, healthy ingredients. Can't have anything really harmful in it' (K7MW-SES3).* The participants selected foods with regard to their medical conditions, modified their eating habits according to physicians' recommendations, allocated more time for meals, endeavoured to eat regularly, consciously managed their body weight and reduced portion sizes. *'We eat at home, three times a day, and pretty much the same stuff every day. What's changed is that we have breakfast calmly and on time. Well, we eat relatively little, I'd say. We definitely eat less' (K5FMar-SES2).*

Other participants explicitly stated that listening to their body was more important. Nevertheless, they were aware that they should monitor their weight. Among some older adults, resilience manifests precisely in the balance between health, pleasure and bodily attunement. The tension between declared freedom and an internal awareness of the need for restraint is also described by Whitelock and Ensaff (2018), who note that food choices were often guided by hedonistic criteria, with sweet and energy-dense foods taking precedence over health considerations. This emphasis on taste emerges as a common characteristic, even though other studies (Andretti et al., 2025; Boles et al., 2022; Kamphuis et al., 2015) indicate that individuals with higher SES typically place greater emphasis on health. In our sample, however, SES did not appear to be a decisive factor in choosing between health-oriented nutrition and pleasure-driven eating: *'As a diabetic, I shouldn't even be eating, I dunno, an apple at five or six o'clock, none of that fruit stuff. But I just say, "Heck, how long am I gonna be here anyway," and I eat it' (K22MD-SES2).*

Bédard et al. (2020) raise an intriguing question regarding whether the enjoyment of food can serve as a tool to support healthy eating. Their review of forty-five studies indicates that enjoyment is associated with sensory experiences, social sharing, dietary variety and mindful eating. Certain dimensions of food enjoyment may thus positively correlate with healthier dietary patterns. However, further research is needed to better understand how enjoyment can be leveraged as a motivating factor to promote health in older adulthood.

In conclusion, it can be affirmed that resilience in eating among older adults develops in the tension between disciplined adherence to healthy eating principles, attentiveness to bodily needs and the pursuit of food-related pleasure. The integration of these three dimensions enables the establishment of a sustainable and meaningful dietary regimen. This balance allows older adults to maintain eating routines that are not only health-promoting but also meaningful and sustainable in everyday life.

5.4 Conclusion

The findings of our qualitative study highlight several key dimensions of resilience. Independence in food-related practices emerges as crucial for maintaining a sense of autonomy and dignity. Gendered practices reveal how deeply everyday activities such as cooking and sharing meals are embedded in cultural norms, and how these roles persist into older age. Mindful eating and the enjoyment of food emphasise that resilience operates not only at a functional level but also at sensory and emotional levels. Adaptation to health limitations and changing life circumstances demonstrates the flexibility of older adults. At the same time, food source diversification and the use of social networks represent concrete strategies for managing structural and environmental barriers. Finally, the knowledge and application of healthy eating principles underscore the importance of information and education in supporting autonomy and health.

In summary, resilience in the eating practices of older adults is not merely a matter of individual choice, it arises from the complex interplay of personal motivation, culturally learned practices and available social and material resources. Understanding these dimensions can contribute to the design of interventions that support healthy and meaningful eating while respecting the needs, traditions and capabilities of older adults.

References

Abbots, E.-J., & Lavis, A. (Eds.). (2016). *Why We Eat, How We Eat: Contemporary Encounters Between Foods and Bodies.* Routledge. https://doi.org/10.4324/9781315547190

Andretti, B., Vieites, Y., Elmor, L., & Andrade, E. B. (2025). How Socioeconomic Status Shapes Food Preferences and Perceptions. *Journal of Marketing*. https://doi.org/10.1177/00222429241296048

Bailly N, Van Wymelbeke V, Maître I, Sulmont-Rossé C. The Assessment of Eating Pleasure among Older Adults: Development and Preliminary Validation of the Anticipatory and Consummatory Eating Pleasure (ACEPS). J Nutr Health Aging. 2020;24(6):606-613. https://doi.org/10.1007/s12603-020-1388-2. PMID: 32510113.

Bédard A, Lamarche PO, Grégoire LM, Trudel-Guy C, Provencher V, Desroches S, Lemieux S. Can eating pleasure be a lever for healthy eating? A systematic scoping review of eating pleasure and its links with dietary behaviors and health. PLoS One. 2020 Dec 21;15(12):e0244292. https://doi.org/10.1371/journal.pone.0244292. PMID: 33347469; PMCID: PMC7751982.

Boles DZ, Turnwald BP, Perry MA, Crum AJ. Emphasizing appeal over health promotes preference for nutritious foods in people of low socioeconomic status. Appetite. 2022 May 1;172:105945. https://doi.org/10.1016/j.appet.2022.105945. Epub 2022 Jan 28. PMID: 35093457.

Bourdieu, P. (1984). Distinction: A Social Critique of the Judgement of Taste. Harvard University Press.

Bowling A, Dieppe P. What is successful ageing and who should define it? BMJ. 2005 Dec 24;331(7531):1548-51. https://doi.org/10.1136/bmj.331.7531.1548. PMID: 16373748; PMCID: PMC1322264.

Brettin, S., Brückner, M., Magnani, N. (2024). A Plate Full of Food and Care: Investigating Care Practices and Gender Relations at the Crossroads of Sustainability, Innovative Practices, and Digital Platforms. In: Dulsrud, A., Forno, F. (eds) Digital Food Provisioning in Times of Multiple Crises. Consumption and Public Life. Palgrave Macmillan, Cham. https://doi.org/10.1007/978-3-031-46323-5_9

Bye, L. M. (2003). Masculinity and rurality at play in stories about hunting. *Norsk Geografisk Tidsskrift - Norwegian Journal of Geography, 57*(3), 145–153. https://doi-org.ezproxy.is.cuni.cz/https://doi.org/10.1080/00291950310002125

Carcedo-Argüelles L, Llamas-Fernández S, Fernández-Álvarez MDM, Caballero-Díaz FF, Rodríguez-Artalejo F, López-García E, Lana A. Sex differences in the association between social frailty and diet quality among older adults in Spain. J Nutr Health Aging. 2024 Oct;28(10):100346. https://doi.org/10.1016/j.jnha.2024.100346. Epub 2024 Aug 26. PMID: 39191117.

Carrière, K., Siemers, N., & Knäuper, B. (2022). A scoping review of mindful eating interventions for obesity management. *Mindfulness, 13*(6), 1387–1402. https://doi.org/10.1007/s12671-022-01883-x

Choi YJ, Crimmins EM, Kim JK, Ailshire JA. Food and nutrient intake and diet quality among older Americans. *Public Health Nutrition.* 2021;24(7):1638-1647. https://doi.org/10.1017/S1368980021000586

Counihan, C. (1999). *The Anthropology of Food and Body: Gender, Meaning and Power*. Routledge.

Dean M, Raats MM, Grunert KG, Lumbers M; Food in Later Life Team. Factors influencing eating a varied diet in old age. Public Health Nutr. 2009 Dec;12(12):2421–7. https://doi.org/10.1017/S1368980009005448. Epub 2009 Apr 6. PMID: 19344544.

DeVault, M. L. (1991). *Feeding the Family: The Social Organization of Caring as Gendered Work.* Chicago: University of Chicago Press. 0226143597; 0226143600

Elo S, Kyngäs H. The qualitative content analysis process. J Adv Nurs. 2008 Apr;62(1):107-15. https://doi.org/10.1111/j.1365-2648.2007.04569.x. PMID: 18352969.

Fischler, C. (1988). Food, self and identity. *Social Science Information, 27*(2), 275-292. https://doi.org/10.1177/053901888027002005 (Original work published 1988)

Folke, C. (2006). Resilience: The emergence of a perspective for social–ecological systems analyses. *Global Environmental Change, 16*(3), 253–267.

Gagnon-Roy M, Pinard S, Bottari C, Le Morellec F, Laliberté C, Ben Lagha R, Yaddaden A, Pigot H, Giroux S, Bier N. Smart Assistive Technology for Cooking for People With Cognitive Impairments Following a Traumatic Brain Injury: User Experience Study. JMIR Rehabil Assist Technol. 2022 Jan 26;9(1):e28701. https://doi.org/10.2196/28701. PMID: 35080496; PMCID: PMC8829699.

GIBAS a kol. (2013): Zahrádkové osady: Stíny minulosti, nebo záblesky budoucnosti. Praha, 147 s. ISBN 978–80–87398–30–2

Goffman, E. (1959). *The Presentation of Self in Everyday Life*. Garden City, NY: Doubleday.

Gough B, Conner MT. Barriers to healthy eating amongst men: a qualitative analysis. Soc Sci Med. 2006 Jan;62(2):387-95. https://doi.org/10.1016/j.socscimed.2005.05.032. Epub 2005 Jul 11. PMID: 16011867.

Hanna K, Cross J, Nicholls A, Gallegos D. The association between loneliness or social isolation and food and eating behaviours: A scoping review. Appetite. 2023 Dec 1;191:107051. https://doi.org/10.1016/j.appet.2023.107051. Epub 2023 Oct 5. PMID: 37802217.

Holtzman, J.D. (2006). Food and Memory. *Annual Review of Anthropology, 35*, 361-378.https://doi.org/10.1146/ANNUREV.ANTHRO.35.081705.123220

Jehlička, Petr, Tomáš Kostelecký, Joe Smith. 2013. „Food Self-Provisioning in Czechia: Beyond Coping Strategy of the Poor: A Response to Alber and Kohler's 'Informal Food Production in the Enlarged European Union' (2008)". *Social Indicators Research.* 111 (1): 219–234. ISSN 0303–8300.

Jensen, T, Grønnow, L, Jespersen, AP. Eating strategies – a qualitative study of how frail, home-dwelling older people in Denmark develop strategies to form meaningful eating situations. *Ageing and Society*. 2019;39(3):590-608. https://doi.org/10.1017/S0144686X17001076

Kamphuis CB, de Bekker-Grob EW, van Lenthe FJ. Factors affecting food choices of older adults from high and low socioeconomic groups: a discrete choice experiment. Am J Clin Nutr. 2015 Apr;101(4):768-74. https://doi.org/10.3945/ajcn.114.096776. Epub 2015 Jan 28. PMID: 25833974.

Kearney MH, Rosal MC, Ockene JK, Churchill LC. Influences on older women's adherence to a low-fat diet in the Women's Health Initiative.

Psychosom Med. 2002 May-Jun;64(3):450–7. https://doi.org/10.1097/00006842-200205000-00009. PMID: 12021418.

Keller HH. Meal programs improve nutritional risk: a longitudinal analysis of community-living seniors. J Am Diet Assoc. 2006 Jul;106(7):1042-8. https://doi.org/10.1016/j.jada.2006.04.023. PMID: 16815120.

Klein L, Parks K. Home Meal Preparation: A Powerful Medical Intervention. Am J Lifestyle Med. 2020 Mar 1;14(3):282-285. https://doi.org/10.1177/1559827620907344. PMID: 32477029; PMCID: PMC7232892.

Locher JL, Ritchie CS, Roth DL, Sen B, Vickers KS, Vailas LI. Food choice among homebound older adults: motivations and perceived barriers. J Nutr Health Aging. 2009 Oct;13(8):659-64. https://doi.org/10.1007/s12603-009-0194-7. PMID: 19657547; PMCID: PMC2749957.

Locher JL, Ritchie CS, Roth DL, Baker PS, Bodner EV, Allman RM. Social isolation, support, and capital and nutritional risk in an older sample: ethnic and gender differences. Soc Sci Med. 2005 Feb;60(4):747-61. https://doi.org/10.1016/j.socscimed.2004.06.023. PMID: 15571893; PMCID: PMC2763304.

Lupton, D. (1996). Food, the body and the self. SAGE Publications Ltd, ISBN 0–8039–7648–8

Macht, M., Meininger, J. & Roth, J. The Pleasures of Eating: A Qualitative Analysis. *J Happiness Stud* 6, 137–160 (2005). https://doi.org/10.1007/s10902-005-0287-x

Mahal ik JR, Burns SM, Syzdek M. Masculinity and perceived normative health behaviors as predictors of men's health behaviors. Soc Sci Med. 2007 Jun;64(11):2201–9. https://doi.org/10.1016/j.socscimed.2007.02.035. Epub 2007 Mar 26. PMID: 17383784.

Mahony LO, Shea EO, O'Connor EM, Tierney A, Harkin M, Harrington J, Kennelly S, Arendt E, O'Toole PW, Timmons S. 'Good, honest food': older adults' and healthcare professionals' perspectives of dietary influences and food preferences in older age in Ireland. J Hum Nutr Diet. 2023 Oct;36(5):1833-1844. https://doi.org/10.1111/jhn.13216. Epub 2023 Jul 31. PMID: 37525412.

Marshall, B. L. (2017). Happily ever after? 'Successful ageing' and the heterosexual imaginary. *European Journal of Cultural Studies, 21*(3), 363-381. https://doi.org/10.1177/1367549417708434 (Original work published 2018)

Middleton G, Patterson KA, Muir-Cochrane E, Velardo S, McCorry F, Coveney J. The Health and Well-being Impacts of Community Shared Meal Programs for Older Populations: A Scoping Review. Innov Aging.

2022 Oct 27;6(7):igac068. https://doi.org/10.1093/geroni/igac068. PMID: 36588625; PMCID: PMC9795837.

Mikkelsen BE. Images of foodscapes: introduction to foodscape studies and their application in the study of healthy eating out-of-home environments. Perspect Public Health. 2011 Sep;131(5):209-16. https://doi.org/10.1177/1757913911415150. PMID: 21999025.

Mol, A. (2021). Eating in Theory. Durham, London: Duke University Press.https://doi.org/10.1215/9781478012924

Moscato Emily M, Julie L. Ozanne; Rebellious eating: older women misbehaving through indulgence. *Qualitative Market Research: An International Journal* 9 September 2019; 22 (4): 582–594. https://doi.org/10.1108/QMR-07-2018-0082

Nyberg, M, Olsson, V, Örtman, G, et al. The meal as a performance: food and meal practices beyond health and nutrition. *Ageing and Society*. 2018;38(1):83-107. https://doi.org/10.1017/S0144686X16000945

Oleschuk, M. (2019). Gender, Cultural Schemas, and Learning to Cook. *Gender & Society*, *33*(4), 607-628. https://doi.org/10.1177/0891243219839669

Oliveira L, Poínhos R, Afonso C, Vaz Almeida MD. Information Sources on Healthy Eating Among Community Living Older Adults. Int Q Community Health Educ. 2021 Jan;41(2):153-158. https://doi.org/10.1177/0272684X20915362. Epub 2020 Apr 4. PMID: 32249704.

Paolini B, Burdette JH, Laurienti PJ, Morgan AR, Williamson DA, Rejeski WJ. Coping with brief periods of food restriction: mindfulness matters. Front Aging Neurosci. 2012 Jun 6;4:13. https://doi.org/10.3389/fnagi.2012.00013. Erratum in: Front Aging Neurosci. 2015 Jan 13;6:345. https://doi.org/10.3389/fnagi.2014.00345. PMID: 22685430; PMCID: PMC3368241.

Payette H, Shatenstein B. Determinants of Healthy Eating in Community-dwelling Elderly People. Can J Public Health. 2005 Jul;96(Suppl 3):S30–5. https://doi.org/10.1007/BF03405198. Epub 2005 Jul 1. PMCID: PMC6976129.13. https://doi.org/10.3389/fnagi.2012.00013

Pixová, M., & Plank, C. (2025). Quiet right to the city: contributing to urban sustainability by converging allotment and community gardens. *Environmental Sociology*, 1–13. https://doi.org/10.1080/23251042.2025.2512599

Plastow NA, Atwal A, Gilhooly M. Food activities and identity maintenance in old age: a systematic review and meta-synthesis. Aging Ment Health. 2015;19(8):667–78. https://doi.org/10.1080/13607863.2014.971707. Epub 2014 Nov 6. PMID: 25373998; PMCID: PMC4440631.

Ramirez-Santos AG, Ravera F, Rivera-Ferre MG, Calvet-Nogués M. Gendered traditional agroecological knowledge in agri-food systems: a systematic review. J Ethnobiol Ethnomed. 2023 Apr 6;19(1):11. https://doi.org/10.1186/s13002-023-00576-6. PMID: 37024903; PMCID: PMC10080974.

Reicks M, Trofholz AC, Stang JS, Laska MN. Impact of cooking and home food preparation interventions among adults: outcomes and implications for future programs. J Nutr Educ Behav. 2014 Jul-Aug;46(4):259–276. https://doi.org/10.1016/j.jneb.2014.02.001. Epub 2014 Apr 1. PMID: 24703245; PMCID: PMC4063875.

Rose L, Wood A, Gill T. Gender differences in adherence and retention in Mediterranean diet interventions with a weight-loss outcome: A systematic review and meta-analysis. Obes Rev. 2024 Dec;25(12):e13824. https://doi.org/10.1111/obr.13824. Epub 2024 Sep 3. PMID: 39228092.

Rueda, S, Artazcoz, L. Gender inequality in health among elderly people in a combined framework of socioeconomic position, family characteristics and social support. *Ageing and Society*. 2009;29(4):625-647. https://doi.org/10.1017/S0144686X08008349

Sachs, C., & Patel-Campillo, A. (2014). Feminist Food Justice: Crafting a New Vision. *Feminist Studies*, *40*(2), 396–410. http://www.jstor.org/stable/https://doi.org/10.15767/feministstudies.40.2.396

Scheper-Hughes, N., & Lock, M. M. (1987). The mindful body: A prolegomenon to future work in medical anthropology. *Medical Anthropology Quarterly*, *1*(1), 6–41. https://doi.org/10.1525/maq.1987.1.1.02a00020

Sellaeg K, Chapman GE. Masculinity and food ideals of men who live alone. Appetite. 2008 Jul;51(1):120-8. https://doi.org/10.1016/j.appet.2008.01.003. Epub 2008 Feb 7. PMID: 18343534.

Seymour-Smith S. Applying discursive approaches to health psychology. Health Psychol. 2015 Apr;34(4):371-80. https://doi.org/10.1037/hea0000165. PMID: 25822053.

Sharkey JR. Diet and health outcomes in vulnerable populations. Ann N Y Acad Sci. 2008;1136:210-7. https://doi.org/10.1196/annals.1425.020. PMID: 18579883.

Sidenvall, B., Nydahl, M., & Fjellström, C. (2000). The Meal as a Gift—The Meaning of Cooking Among Retired Women. *Journal of Applied Gerontology*, *19*(4), 405-423. https://doi.org/10.1177/073346480001900403 (Original work published 2000)

Sivri D, Yur F (2024) Determination of Nutritional Status and Mindful Eating of Elderly Individuals. J Food Sci Nutr 10: 202. https://doi.org/10.24966/FSN-1076/100202

Tani Y, Fujiwara T, Kondo K. Cooking skills related to potential benefits for dietary behaviors and weight status among older Japanese men and women: a cross-sectional study from the JAGES. Int J Behav Nutr Phys Act. 2020 Jun 26;17(1):82. https://doi.org/10.1186/s12966-020-00986-9. PMID: 32590984; PMCID: PMC7318755.

Tucher EL, Keeney T, Cohen AJ, Thomas KS. Conceptualizing Food Insecurity Among Older Adults: Development of a Summary Indicator in the National Health and Aging Trends Study. J Gerontol B Psychol Sci Soc Sci. 2021 Nov 15;76(10):2063-2072. https://doi.org/10.1093/geronb/gbaa147. PMID: 33001172; PMCID: PMC8599055.

Twigg, J. (2004). The body, gender, and age: Feminist insights in social gerontology. *Journal of Aging Studies*, 18(1), 59–73. https://doi.org/10.1016/j.jaging.2003.09.001

Twigg J. (2013). Fashion and Age. Dress, the Body and Later Life. London: Bloomsbury, ISBN 978 1 8748 8696 5

Veen, E. J. B., B. Bock, W. Van den Berg, A. J. Visser & J. S. C. Wiskerke (2015):Community gardening and social cohesion: different designs, different motivations, LocalEnvironment, https://doi.org/10.1080/13549839.2015.1101433

Vesnaver E, Keller HH, Sutherland O, Maitland SB, Locher JL. Alone at the table: Food behavior and the loss of commensality in widowhood. J Gerontol B Psychol Sci Soc Sci. 2016 Nov;71(6):1059–1069. https://doi.org/10.1093/geronb/gbv103. Epub 2015 Nov 10. PMID: 26556790; PMCID: PMC6083990.

Vesnaver E, Keller HH, Payette H, Shatenstein B. Dietary resilience as described by older community-dwelling adults from the NuAge study "if there is a will -there is a way!". Appetite. 2012 Apr;58(2):730-8. https://doi.org/10.1016/j.appet.2011.12.008. Epub 2011 Dec 16. PMID: 22200412.

Vesnaver E, Keller HH. Social influences and eating behavior in later life: a review. J Nutr Gerontol Geriatr. 2011;30(1):2-23. https://doi.org/10.1080/01639366.2011.545038. PMID: 23286638.

Walker, A. and Maltby, T. (2012), Active ageing: A strategic policy solution to demographic ageing in the European Union. International Journal of Social Welfare, 21: S117-S130. https://doi.org/10.1111/j.1468-2397.2012.00871.x

Wang X, Qi J, Zhang K, Xie H, Wu X. The joy of eating: how eating experiences enhance the well-being of older adults. Front Public Health. 2024 Sep 9;12:1438964. https://doi.org/10.3389/fpubh.2024.1438964. PMID: 39314795; PMCID: PMC11417023.

Whitelock E, Ensaff H. On Your Own: Older Adults' Food Choice and Dietary Habits. Nutrients. 2018 Mar 27;10(4):413. https://doi.org/10.3390/nu10040413. PMID: 29584644; PMCID: PMC5946198.
Wiles JL, Wild K, Kerse N, Allen RES. Resilience from the point of view of older people: 'There's still life beyond a funny knee'. Soc Sci Med. 2012 Feb;74(3):416-424. https://doi.org/10.1016/j.socscimed.2011.11.005. Epub 2011 Dec 14. PMID: 22204841.
Wills, W., Backett-Milburn, K., Roberts, M.-L., & Lawton, J. (2011). The Framing of Social Class Distinctions through Family Food and Eating Practices. *The Sociological Review, 59*(4), 725-740. https://doi.org/10.1111/j.1467-954X.2011.02035.x (Original work published 2011)
Winkens LHH, van Strien T, Barrada JR, Brouwer IA, Penninx BWJH, Visser M. The Mindful Eating Behavior Scale: Development and Psychometric Properties in a Sample of Dutch Adults Aged 55 Years and Older. J Acad Nutr Diet. 2018 Jul;118(7):1277-1290.e4. https://doi.org/10.1016/j.jand.2018.01.015. Epub 2018 Apr 11. PMID: 29655657.
Xu, Z., Bao, Y., Dong, H. *et al.* Heart of the future home: a multidimensional model of inclusive kitchen for older people in the UK. *Humanit Soc Sci Commun* 11, 990 (2024). https://doi.org/10.1057/s41599-024-03508-1
Yin Z, Brasher MS, Kraus VB, Lv Y, Shi X, Zeng Y. Dietary Diversity Was Positively Associated with Psychological Resilience among Elders: A Population-Based Study. Nutrients. 2019 Mar 18;11(3):650. https://doi.org/10.3390/nu11030650. PMID: 30889808; PMCID: PMC6471509.

6

General Discussion and Conclusion

Abstract This chapter presents a summary of the findings from a qualitative study that explored how older adults in the Czech Republic develop dietary resilience strategies. Based on qualitative research using semi-structured interviews, the findings demonstrate that everyday food practices are shaped not only by biological needs but also lifelong cultural norms, gender roles and social relationships. The analysis revealed several key dimensions of resilience: the significance of autonomy and self-sufficiency, gendered eating patterns, mindful eating and the joy of food, adaptation to health limitations and life changes, food source diversification and reliance on social networks, as well as the role of nutritional knowledge and education. The study emphasises that resilience is not solely an individual capacity but is embedded in the interplay between personal motivation, culturally acquired practices and available social and material resources. The results thus contribute to a deeper understanding of ageing as a culturally mediated experience and, at the same time, point to practical pathways for supporting a dignified and high-quality in later adulthood.

Keywords Resilience · Eating · Ageing · Food anthropology · Gender · Quality of life · Cultural practices

E. Ferrarová, *Dietary Resilience Strategies in Older Adults with Physical Disabilities*,
https://doi.org/10.1007/978-3-032-22186-5_6

6.1 General Discussion

This book explores the significance of food for older adults, their eating patterns and the resilience strategies and mechanisms they develop in response to changes in health status, socioeconomic circumstances and cultural context. Nutrition among older adults is receiving increasing attention due to demographic forecasts of an ageing global population. Questions concerning quality of life have become a priority, and this includes food, which forms the foundation not only of biological but also psychological wellbeing. Food is essential for survival, yet it also represents a source of pleasure and a way of maintaining or improving health. It also provides older adults with much-needed structure, continuity and autonomy. This book contributes to the current discussion on older adults' nutrition.

The development of resilience strategies and mechanisms in the eating practices of older adults is a dynamic and multilayered process that connects individual resources, social ties and cultural practices. This process is not isolated but embedded in broader structural conditions, such as socioeconomic inequalities, gender roles and access to healthcare. Theoretical frameworks of resilience (Windle, 2011; Ungar, 2012) show that resilience is not an individual's static trait but a negotiation process between personal capacities and environmental conditions. The empirical findings of this study support this perspective. Although older adults face challenges such as retirement, health limitations, widowhood or social isolation, they are able to maintain a sense of continuity and meaning by developing strategies rooted in cultural norms and daily routines.

The qualitative research presented in this book is based on interviews and observations of community-dwelling older adults, aiming to clarify the extent to which they can mobilise resources that enable them to develop and apply dietary strategies, thereby preserving continuity in eating and creating meaningful eating situations (Whitelock & Ensaff, 2018). The study found that eating resilience is a lived experience, not an abstract concept. The value of a qualitative approach lies in its ability to capture the nuances of everyday life—for example, the significance of small adaptive steps, the importance of commensality or the ways in which people combine expert recommendations with their own preferences and routines. This methodological perspective highlights the importance of older adults' subjective experience and demonstrates that resilience unfolds within the context of daily decisions and relationships, which quantitative approaches often cannot fully capture.

The empirical research showed that a key motivational factor in the development of resilience strategies is the effort to maintain health and autonomy, as also documented in previous studies (Vesnaver & Keller, 2011). Maintaining good health was explicitly mentioned by the majority of participants, with knowledge of health limitations and the ability to adapt their diet accordingly being crucial. At the same time, it emerged that resistance to recommendations can also be an expression of resilience—an act through which older adults assert their independence. This ambivalence confirms that resilience cannot be reduced to 'good' or 'bad' strategies but should be understood as a process reflecting individual choices, cultural patterns and structural conditions.

When motivated, resilience strategies can emerge, the most important of which were identified as mindful eating and enjoyment of food, adapting diet to changes, diversifying food sources, creating supportive social networks and adhering to healthy eating principles.

In our sample, 14 of 23 participants reported applying the principle of mindful eating and seeking pleasure from food. Although the significance of enjoyment in eating varies across cultures, experts agree that food-related pleasure in this demographic can help prevent or overcome food-related apathy resulting from health limitations and illness (Locher et al., 2009). Our findings also show that, for community-dwelling older adults, social interaction during meals or fine dining is not necessarily a priority. Instead, older adults tend to mobilise resources to create strategies that allow them to shape a dining environment they consider good and manageable, where they can engage in activities that support their own perceptions and desires regarding wellbeing in eating.

Specific patterns were identified that may illuminate the interpretation of adaptive and resilience mechanisms in eating, as well as strategies aimed at maintaining dignified and independent nutrition even in the presence of health limitations or impairments. Observed creative approaches among the participants included maintaining and developing social ties and creating alternatives to previous eating habits, with the goal of preserving quality of life and health. Knowledge of food and nutrition, cooking skills, sufficient financial resources and support from family, friends and neighbours facilitated the development of resilience strategies to overcome nutritional vulnerability. For participants, the ability to continue eating in a way that made sense to them was more important than socially established food preparation and consumption rules.

Another significant finding is the gendered nature of eating practices. Differences between men and women in nutrition are not a matter of biological predispositions but stem from long-standing social roles and cultural expectations. The differing strategies of men and women are firmly rooted in daily practices (Carcedo-Argüelles et al., 2024). Among older adults, the relationship to one's body is also gendered, serving as a measure through which resilience becomes visible: from weight regulation to mindful eating and food-related pleasure.

The findings also indicate that eating among older adults should be understood not merely as an individual choice, but primarily as a process embedded in social relationships, cultural norms and the changing conditions of life in old age. In this sense, dietary resilience emerges as a concept linking individual adaptability with the sociocultural and material conditions that influence ageing and everyday food practices.

6.2 Conclusion

A novel contribution of this work to the study of older adults' eating lies in connecting food anthropology with gerontological theories, which makes it possible to approach ageing not only as a biological process but also as a culturally shaped experience.

The research results show that lifelong family patterns, gendered perceptions and eating habits significantly influence older adults' dietary strategies. In particular, the development of strategies related to body perception illustrates gender-conditioned eating patterns among older adults. On this basis, it is suggested that any analysis of older adults' dietary needs should always include a gender perspective, as this enables a deeper understanding of the resources mobilised in relation to eating strategies.

Findings also confirmed that motivation is crucial for the creation of resilience strategies, as older adults view food as the key to their health and independence. However, even with strong motivation, individuals may be constrained by the resources available to them. Assessing personal food-related resources is therefore essential for determining an individual's capacity to be resilient. The research shows that when personal resources are insufficient, older adults must be willing to rely on both informal and formal support. Yet many older people resist dependence on others, perceiving it as a sign of ageing and a loss of autonomy and control. Caregivers and healthcare professionals may need to address these attitudes and help individuals in their care to understand that support is sometimes necessary in order to achieve their goals. At the same time, older adults' interest in food as a key to dignified ageing can be strengthened by reinforcing the belief that food and food-related activities may serve as a source of pleasure and joy.

6.2.1 Implications and Future Research

The results of this book have both practical and research implications. On the practical level, they show that supporting dignified ageing through food should not be reduced merely to nutritional recommendations but should also encompass cultural meanings and gender differences. Programmes aimed at older adults should more fully reflect their social roles, daily routines and the ways in which food retains its symbolic significance despite health limitations. Practical steps may include:

- educational campaigns focused on nutritional literacy and informed food choices,
- support for communal dining and collective cooking as tools against isolation and

- gender-sensitive programmes that take into account the specific needs of different groups (e.g., men who begin cooking for themselves after being widowed).

Such interventions can contribute not only to a better quality of life for individuals but also to strengthening resilience at the community level.

Another challenge in the eating practices of older adults is the prevalence of large food packages and oversized portions in food services. Smaller portions at lower prices could better suit reduced appetite as well as financial considerations. Smaller portions in gastronomy and smaller packaging by food retailers also have the potential to reduce food waste, improve dietary diversity and expand consumer choice. These adjustments would simultaneously represent institutional support for resilience, as they would make it easier for older people to choose meals that match their needs and circumstances.

Although the qualitative approach provided deep insight into the individual experiences of older people, the results of this study cannot be generalised to the entire population. The sample size and its cultural embeddedness represent limitations that must be considered. In the future, combining qualitative and quantitative approaches is desirable so as to connect individual perspectives with broader population data.

Another direction is international comparison, which would allow different cultural contexts to be contrasted and reveal the extent to which resilience strategies are universal or culturally specific. Longitudinal studies capturing changes in dietary strategies and their relationship to shifting life circumstances would also be useful. Finally, more attention should be paid to the intersection of gender, socioeconomic status and educational attainment since their interaction significantly shapes the form and effectiveness of resilience strategies.

Food in later life is not merely a matter of nutrition but represents a deeply rooted cultural and social practice through which identity, gender roles and the ability to cope with change and loss are shaped. Dietary resilience in older adults emerges as a dynamic process in which biological, psychological and sociocultural dimensions intertwine. It thus contributes not only to understanding individual experiences of ageing but also to creating supportive environments that can appreciate the significance of food for quality of life.

In closing, this book also opens space for further discussion and research challenging the perception that eating is solely a daily necessity and repositioning it as a source of meaning, connection, strength and pleasure in later life.

References

Carcedo-Argüelles L, Llamas-Fernández S, Fernández-Álvarez MDM, Caballero-Díaz FF, Rodríguez-Artalejo F, López-García E, Lana A. Sex differences in the association between social frailty and diet quality among older adults in Spain. J Nutr Health Aging. 2024 Oct;28(10):100346. https://doi.org/10.1016/j.jnha.2024.100346. Epub 2024 Aug 26. PMID: 39191117.

Locher JL, Ritchie CS, Roth DL, Sen B, Vickers KS, Vailas LI. Food choice among homebound older adults: motivations and perceived barriers. J Nutr Health Aging. 2009 Oct;13(8):659-64. https://doi.org/10.1007/s12603-009-0194-7. PMID: 19657547; PMCID: PMC2749957.

Ungar, M. (Ed.). (2012). *The social ecology of resilience: A handbook of theory and practice.* Springer Science + Business Media. https://doi.org/10.1007/978-1-4614-0586-3

Vesnaver E, Keller HH. Social influences and eating behavior in later life: a review. J Nutr Gerontol Geriatr. 2011;30(1):2-23. https://doi.org/10.1080/01639366.2011.545038. PMID: 23286638.

Whitelock E, Ensaff H. On Your Own: Older Adults' Food Choice and Dietary Habits. Nutrients. 2018 Mar 27;10(4):413. https://doi.org/10.3390/nu10040413. PMID: 29584644; PMCID: PMC5946198.

Windle, G. (2011). What is resilience? A review and concept analysis. *Reviews in Clinical Gerontology, 21*(2), 152–169. https://doi.org/10.1017/S0959259810000420

Index

E. Ferrarová, *Dietary Resilience Strategies in Older Adults with Physical Disabilities*,
https://doi.org/10.1007/978-3-032-22186-5

FSC
www.fsc.org
MIX
Papier | Fördert
gute Waldnutzung
FSC® C083411

Kolibri 360 GmbH
Ferdinand-Jühlke-Straße 7
99095 Erfurt, Deutschland
produktsicherheit@kolibri360.de